EASY ADULT COLORING BOOK

Ocean Life

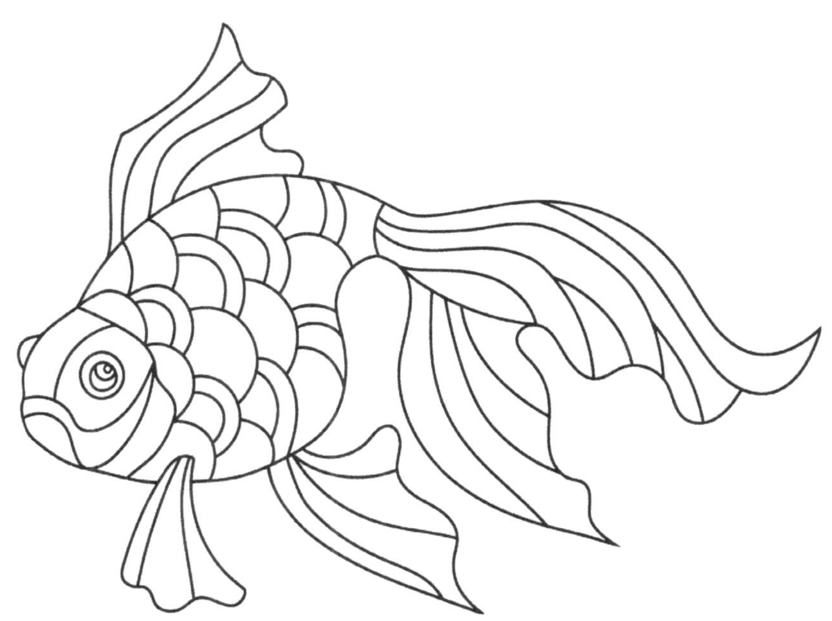

Love Yourself

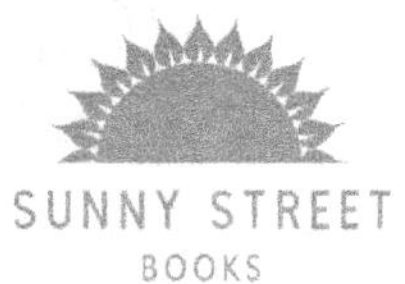
SUNNY STREET
BOOKS

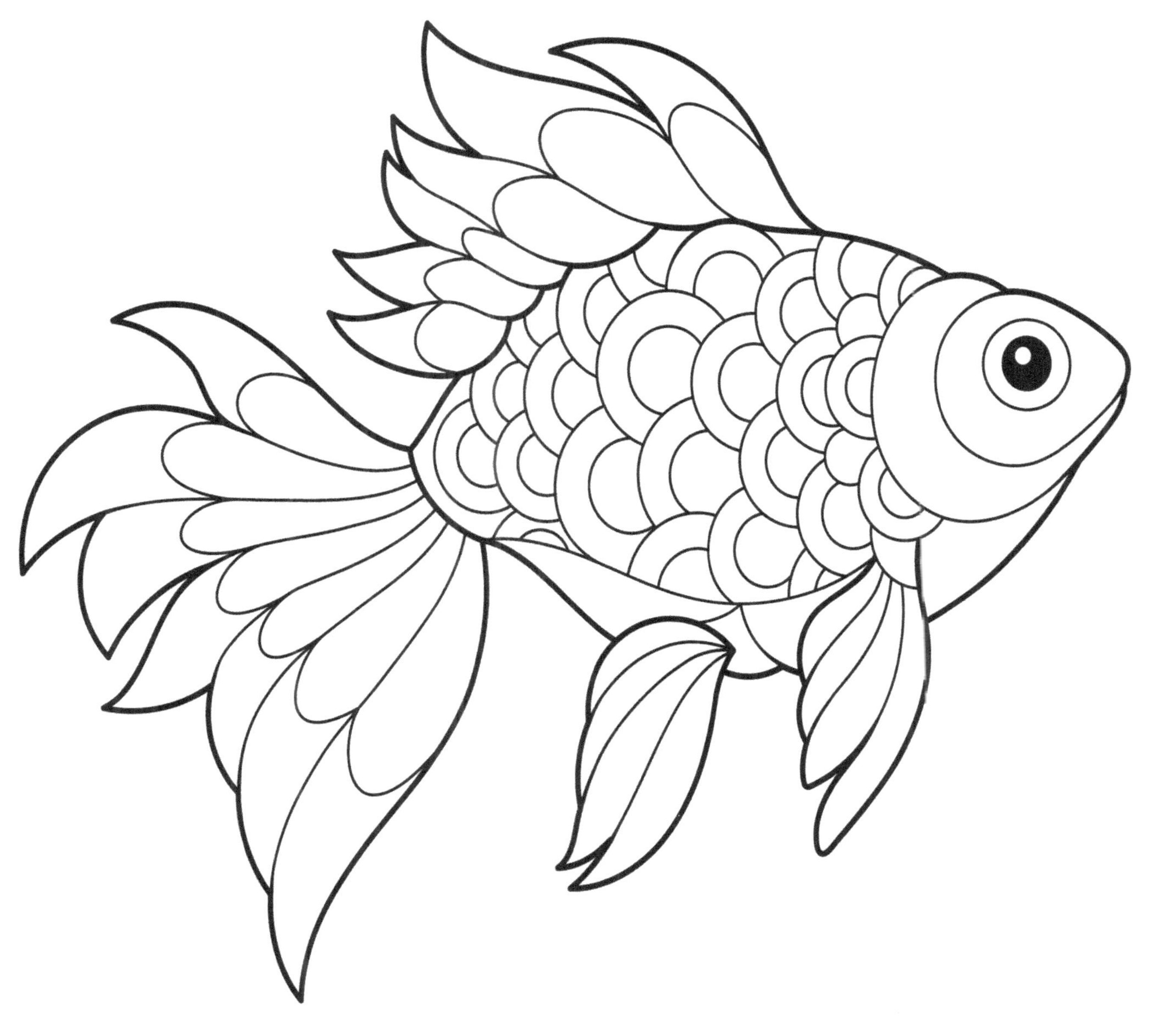

Always Calm

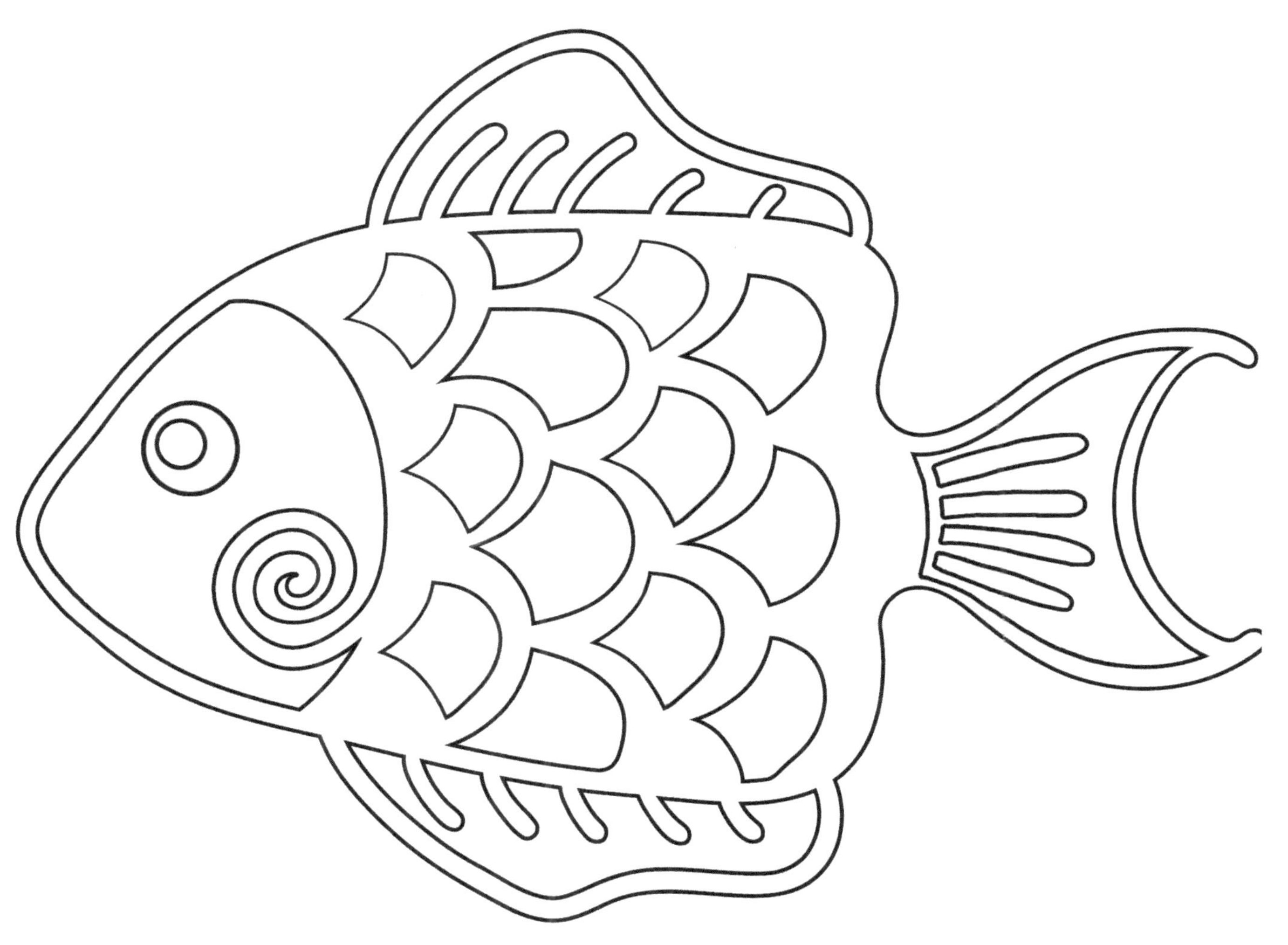

Be Brave

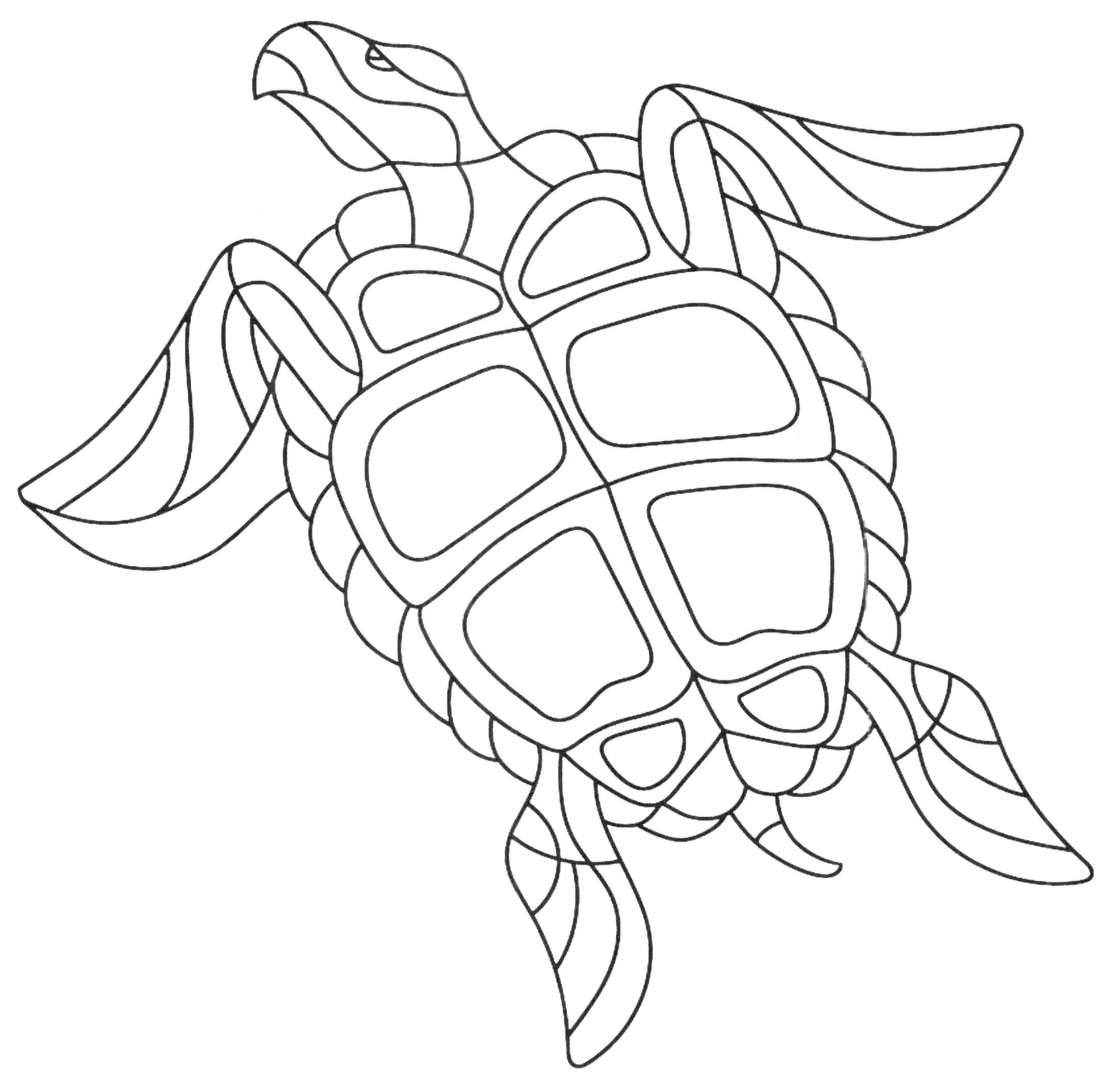

Be Fearless

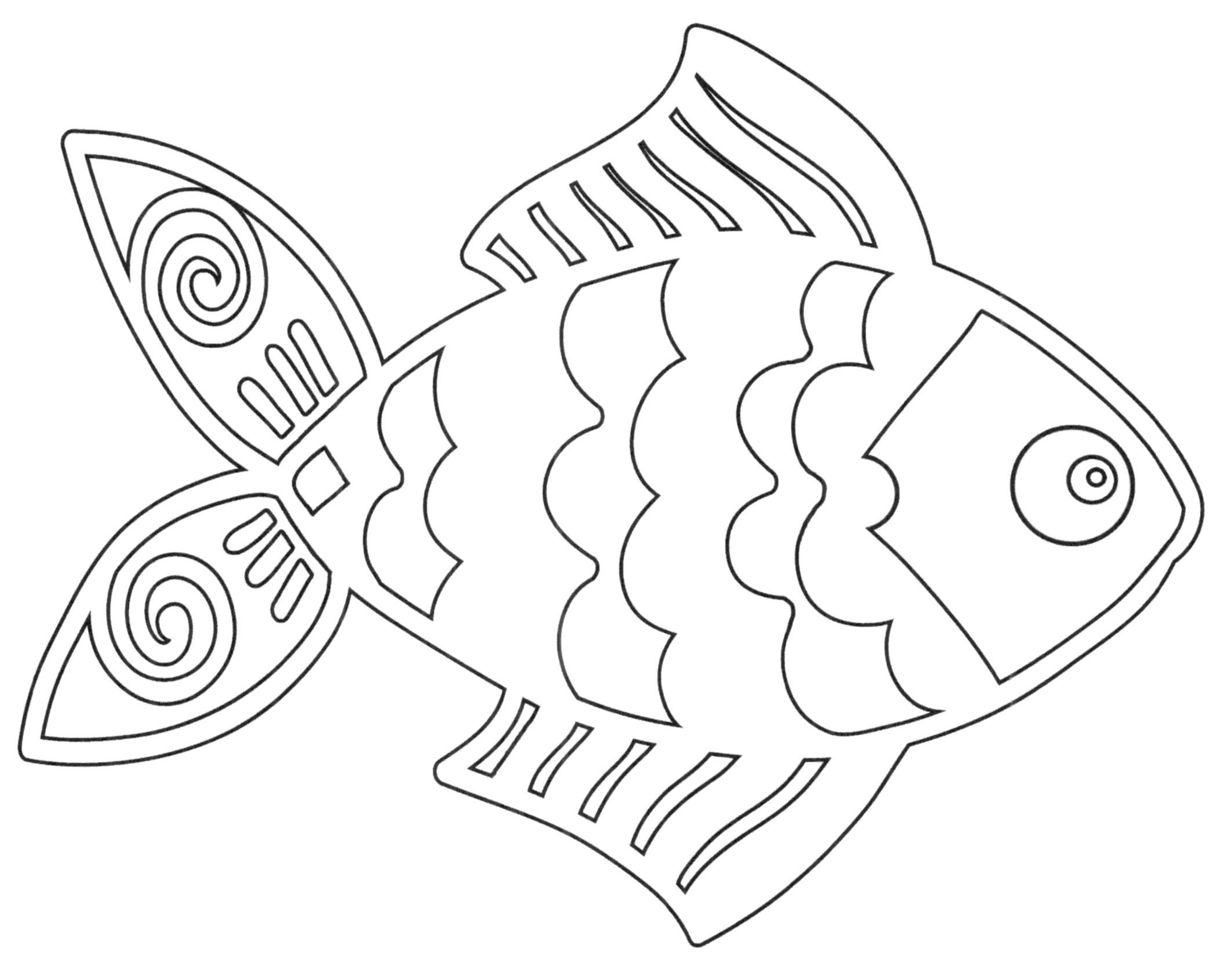

Be Happy

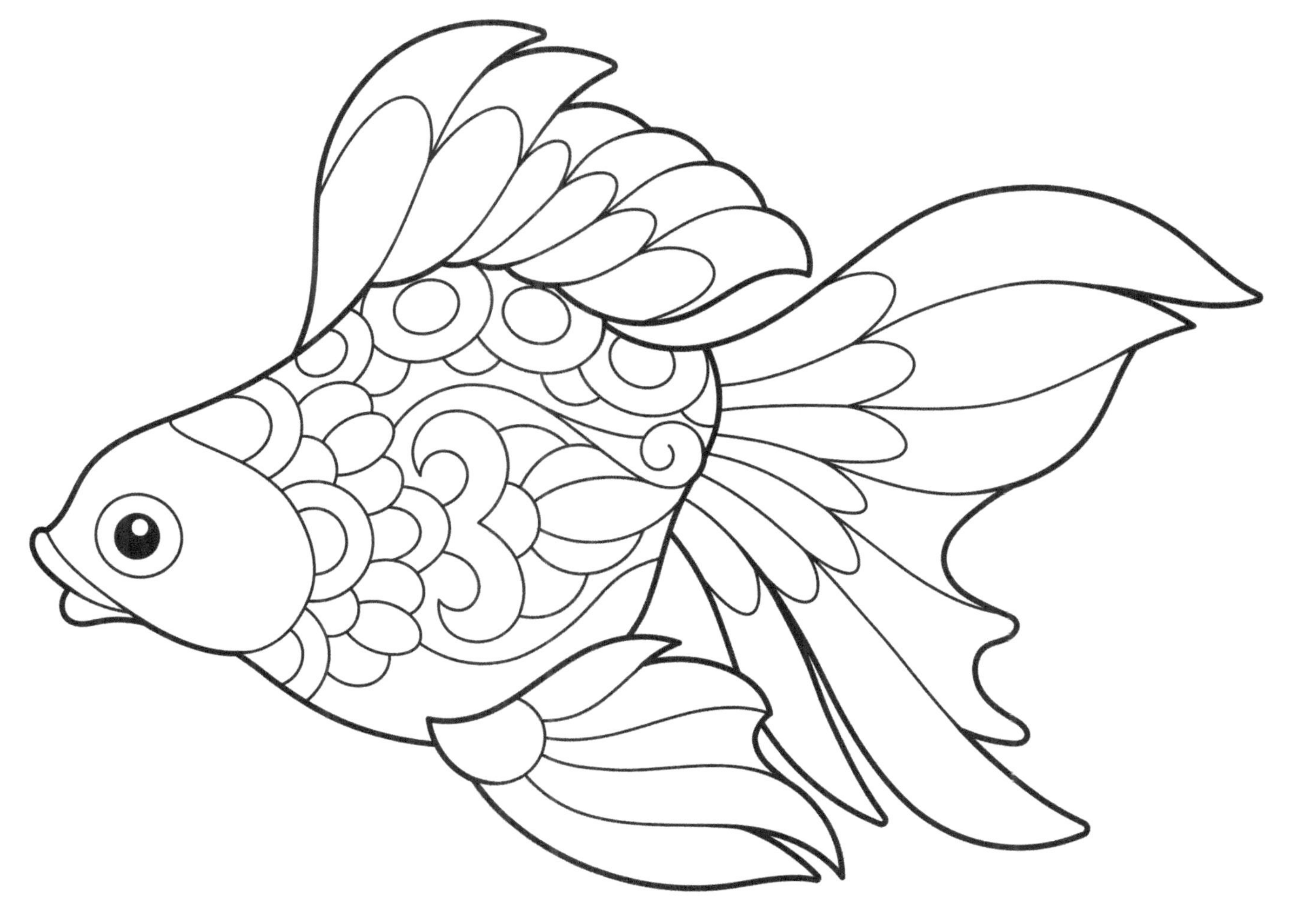

Be Kind

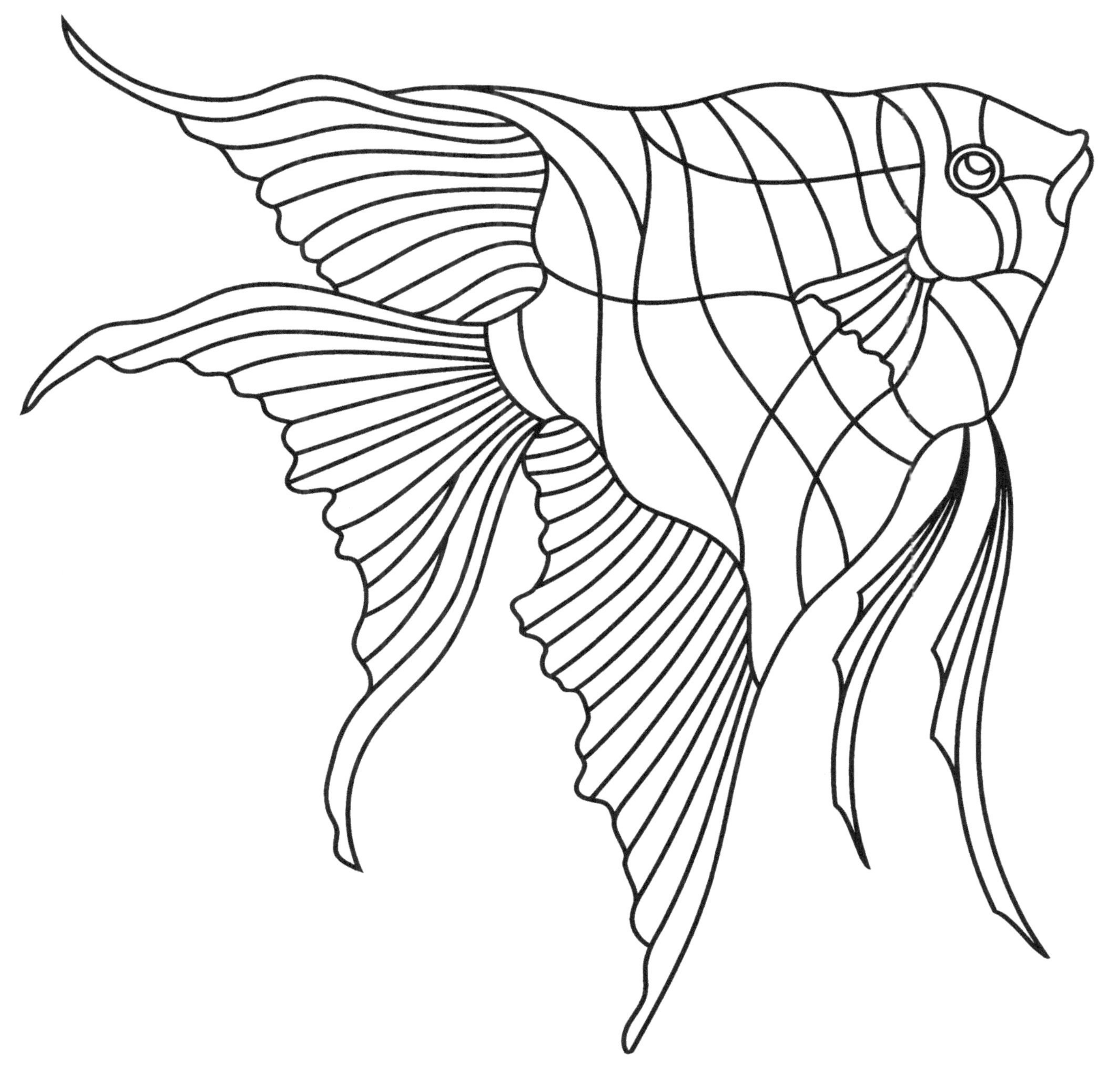

Bless You

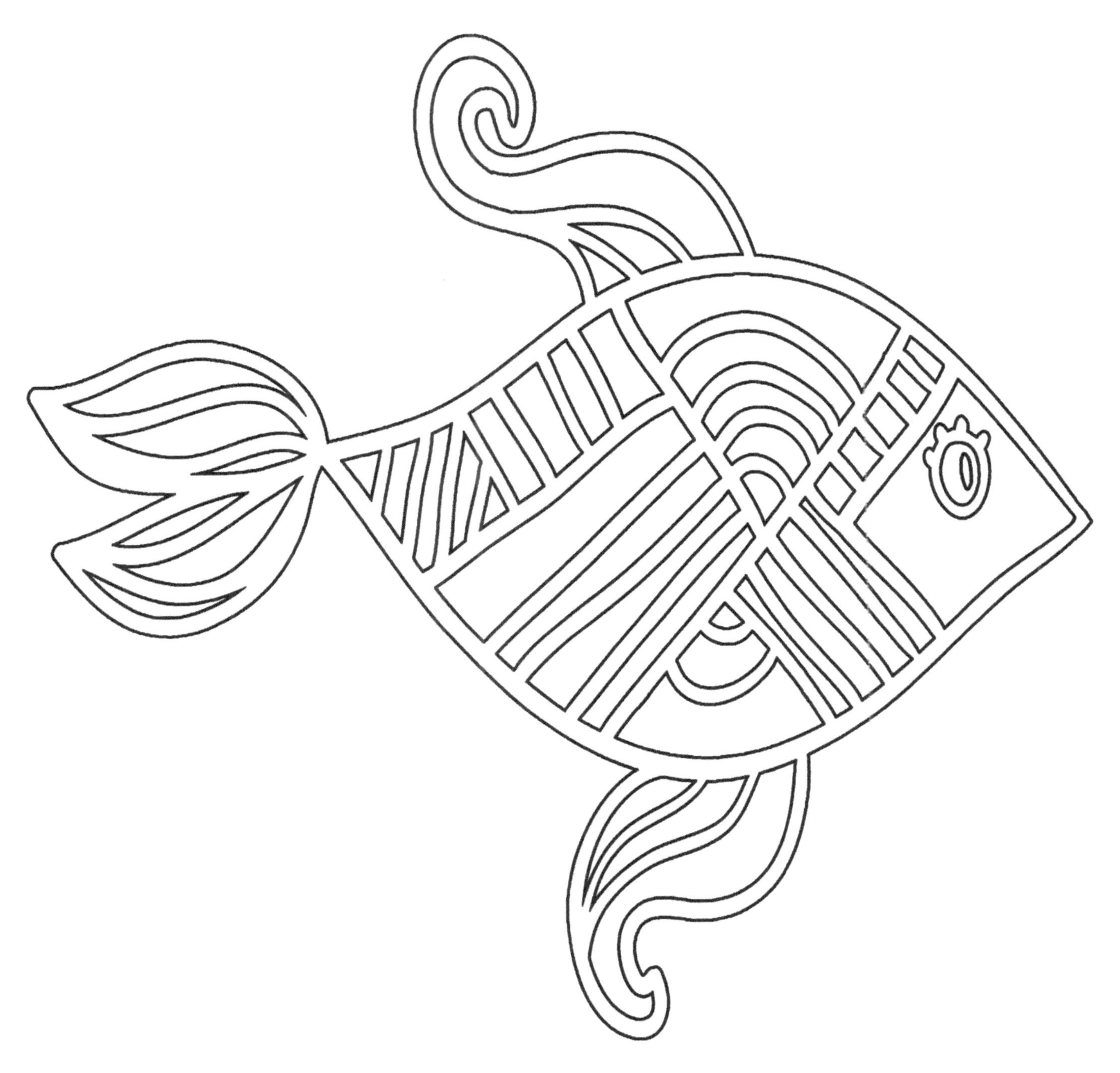

Breathe Deeply

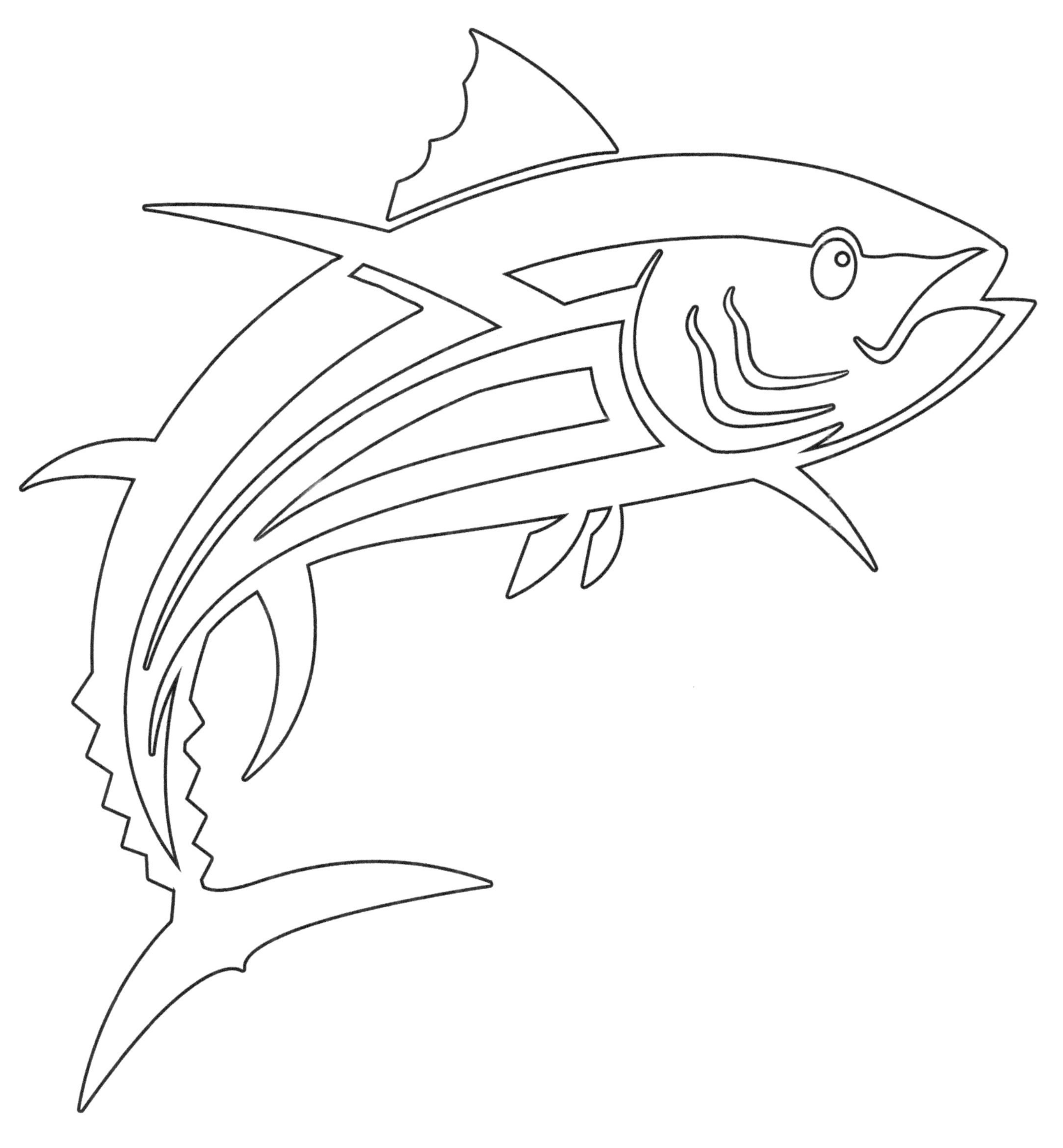

Cherish Today

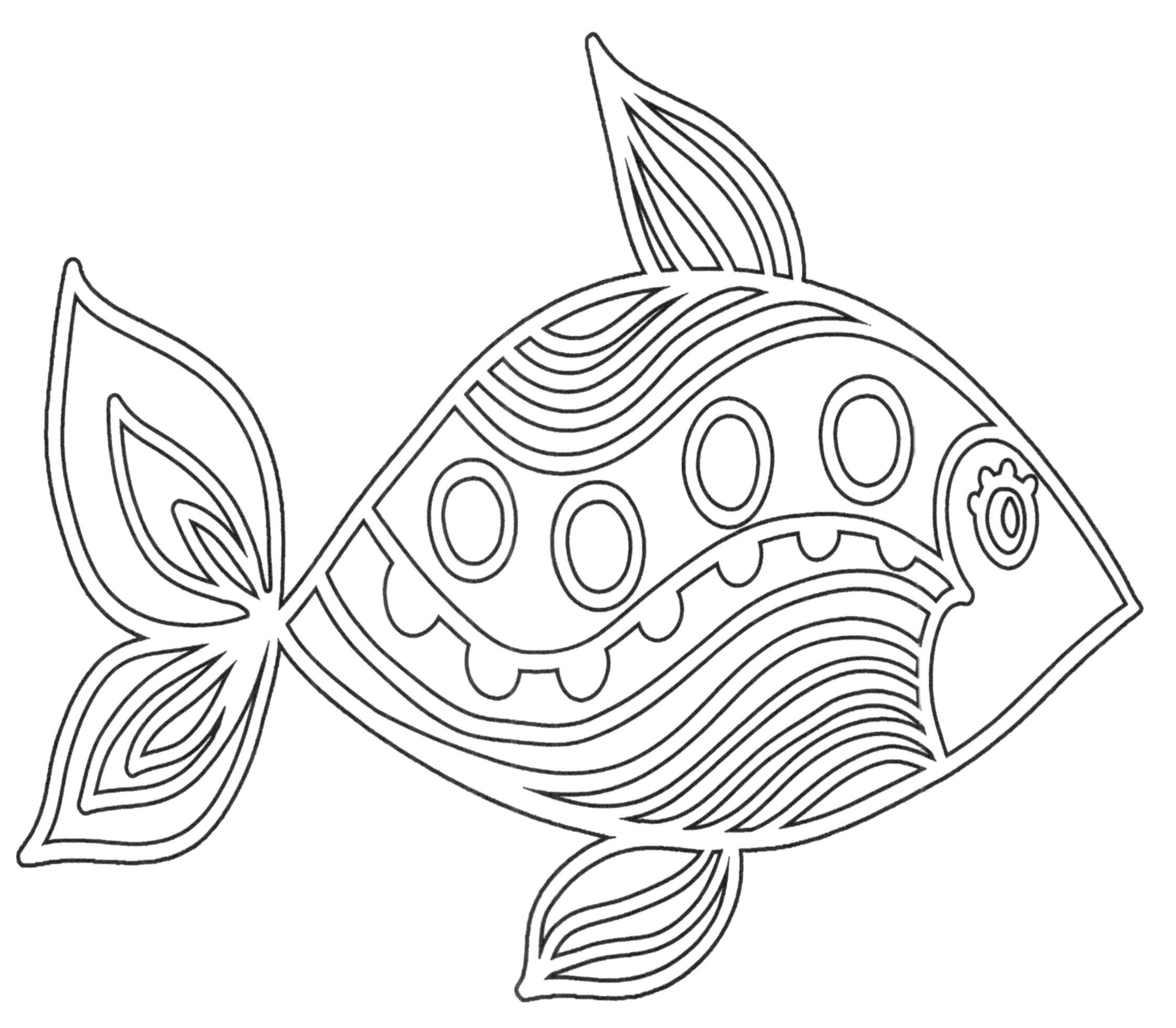

Dream Big

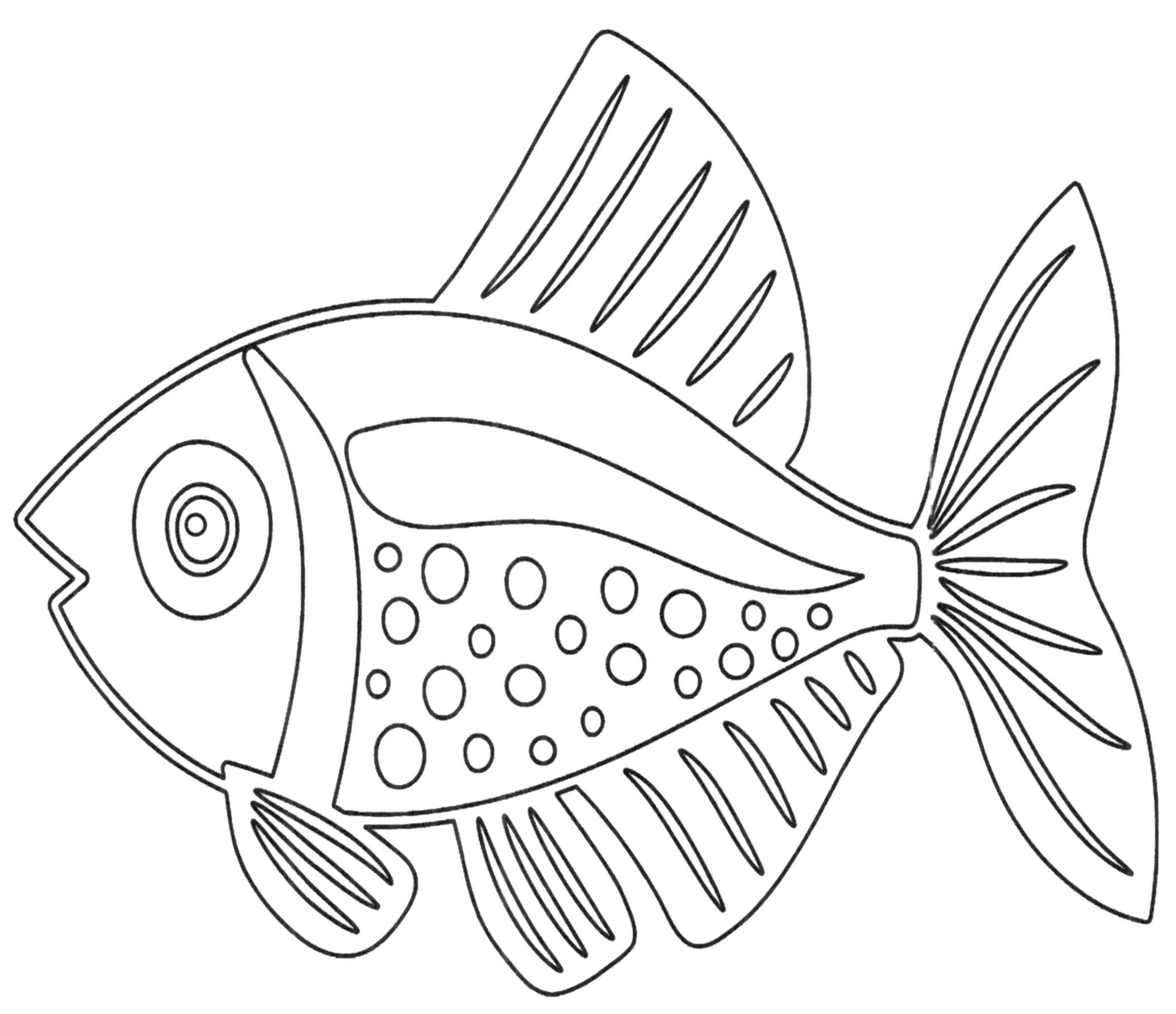

Enjoy Life

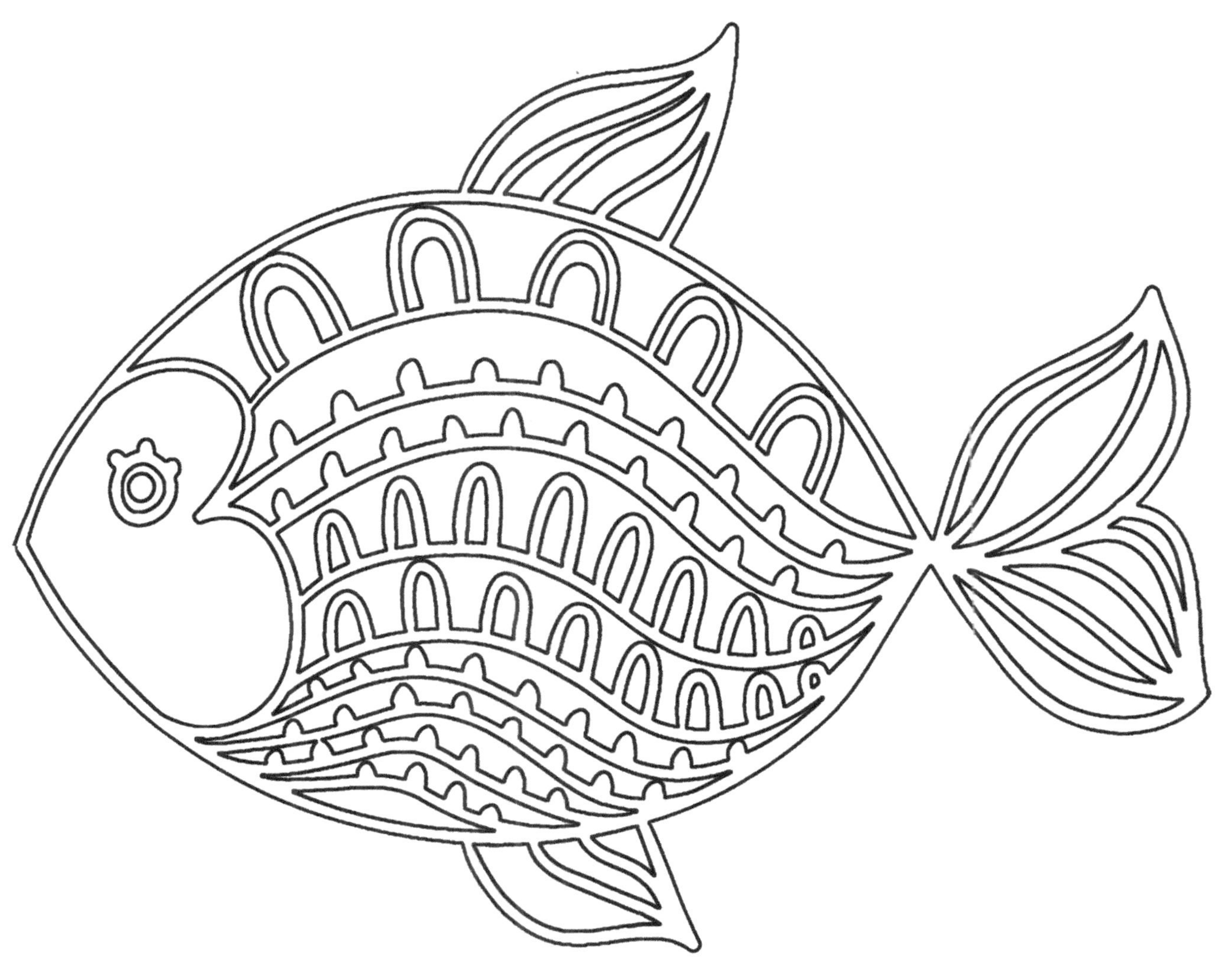

Eternal Sunshine

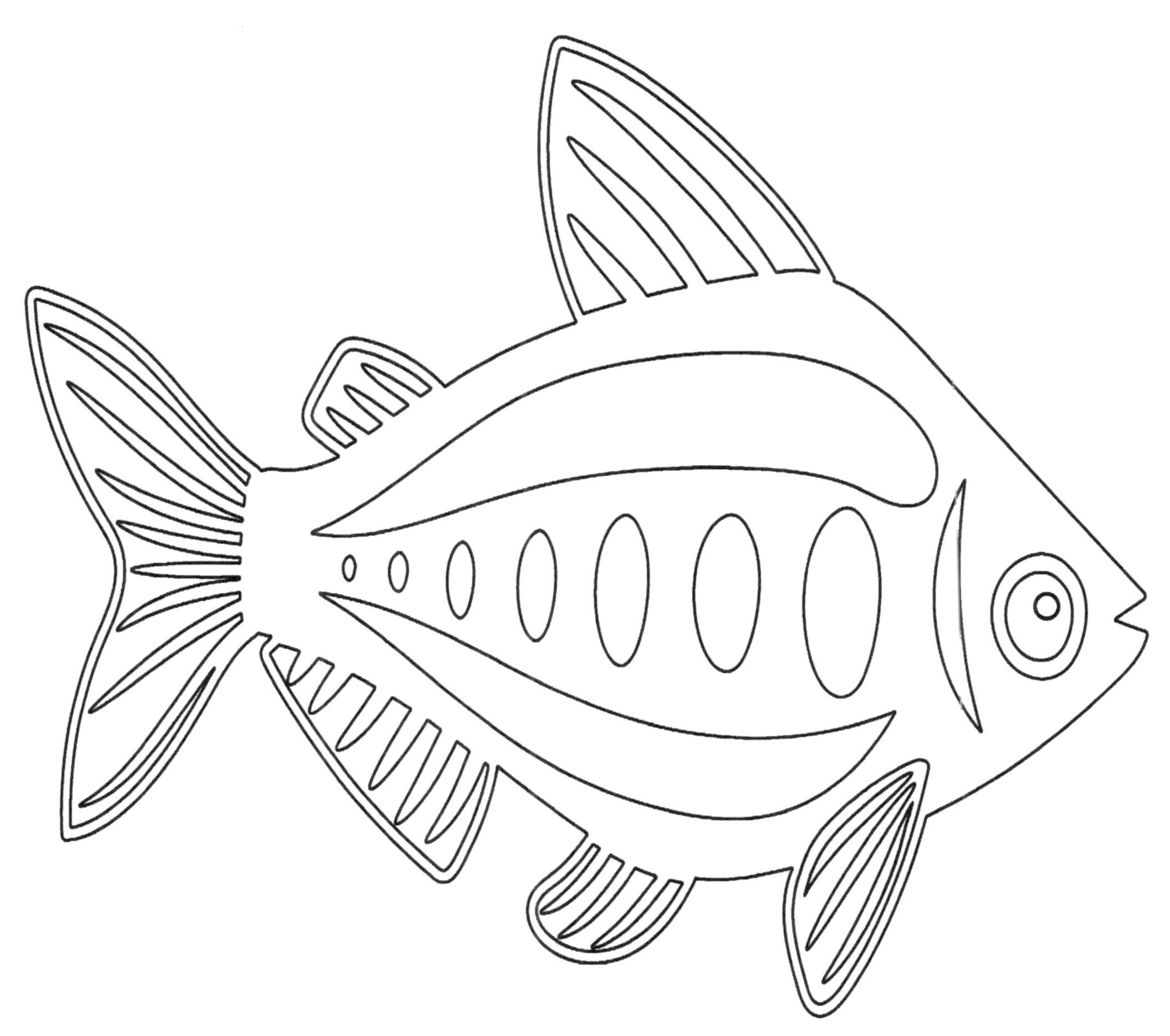

Fear Not

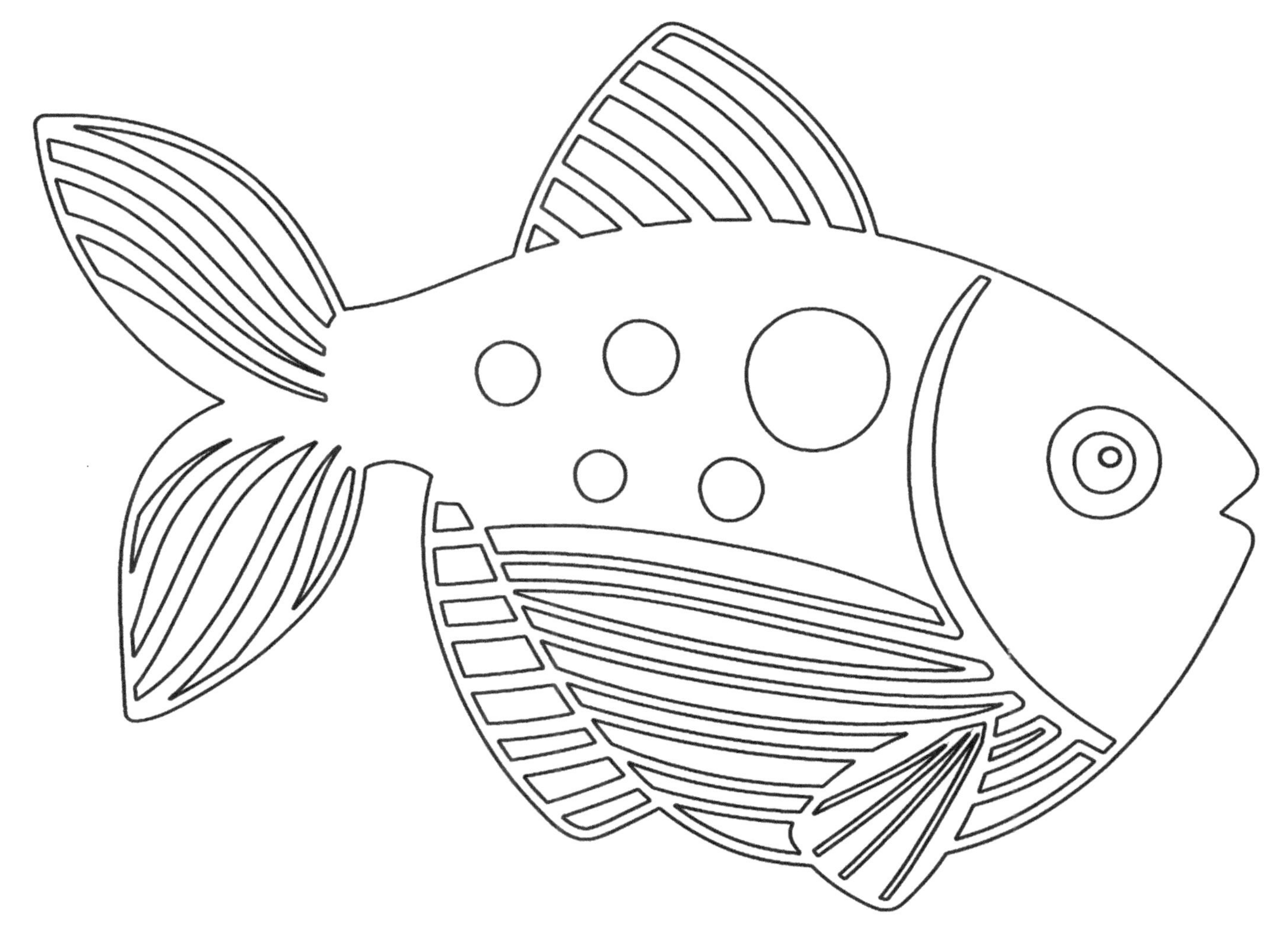

Find Balance

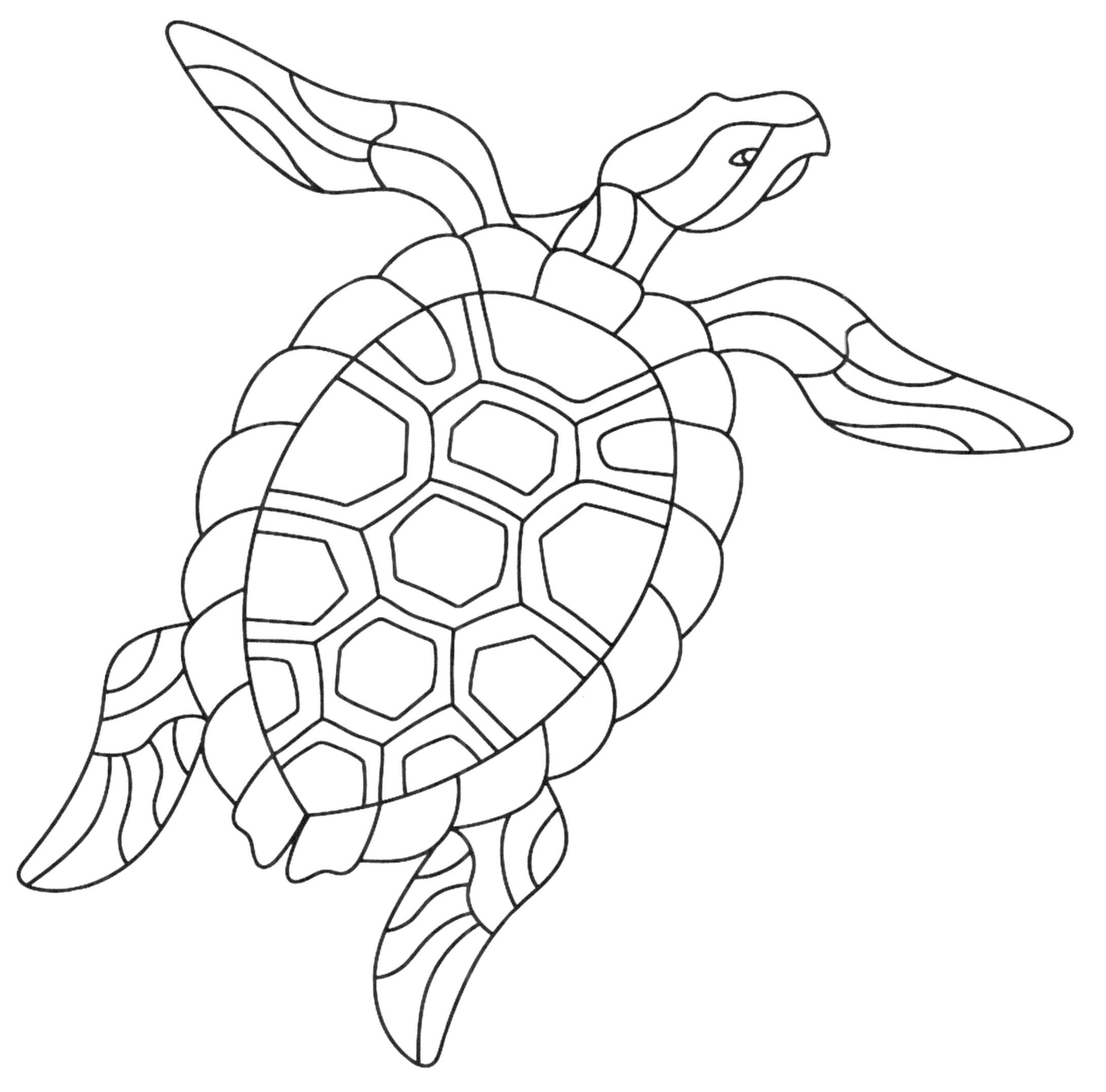

Forever Free

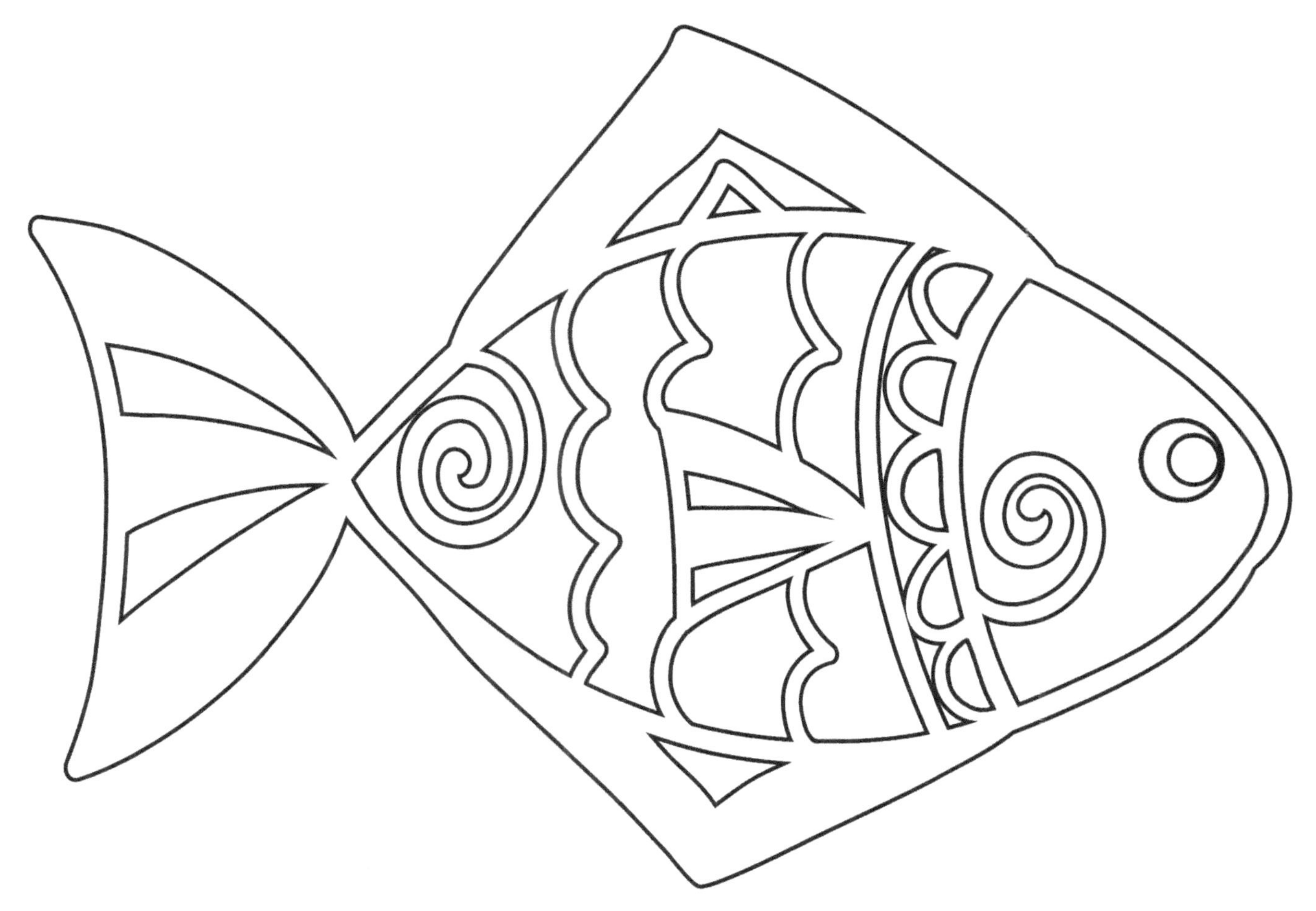

Friends Forever

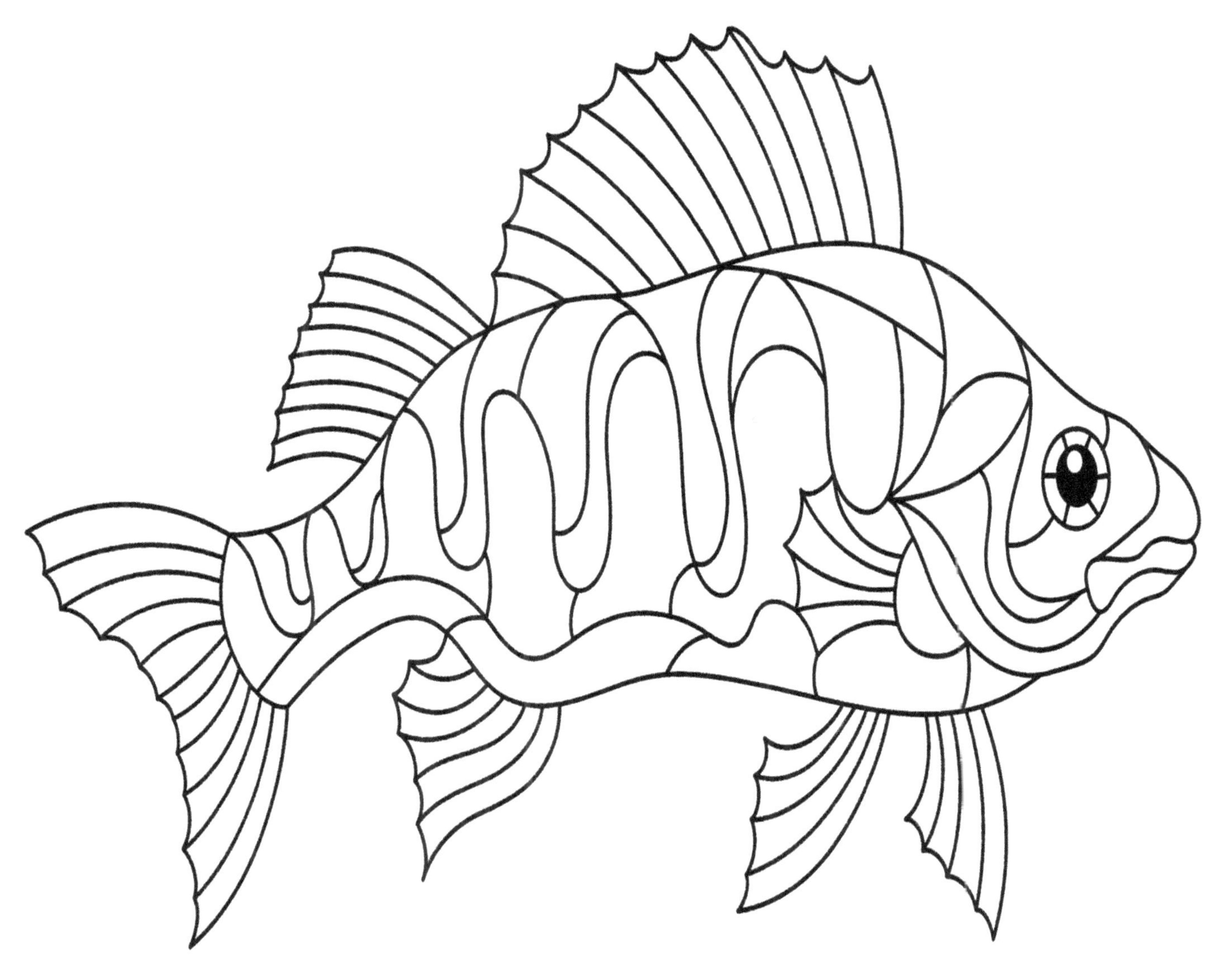

Give Thanks

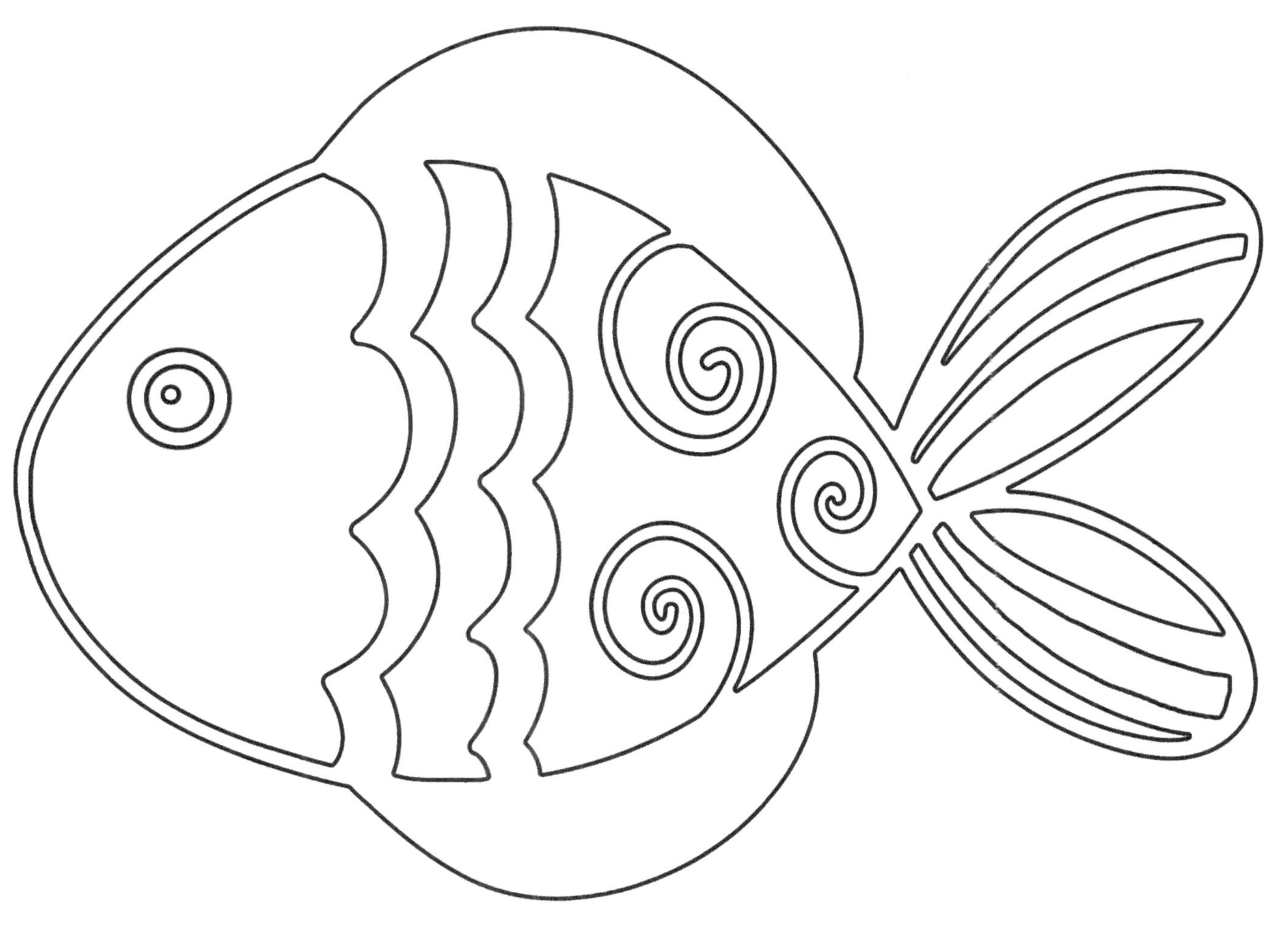

Happy Endings

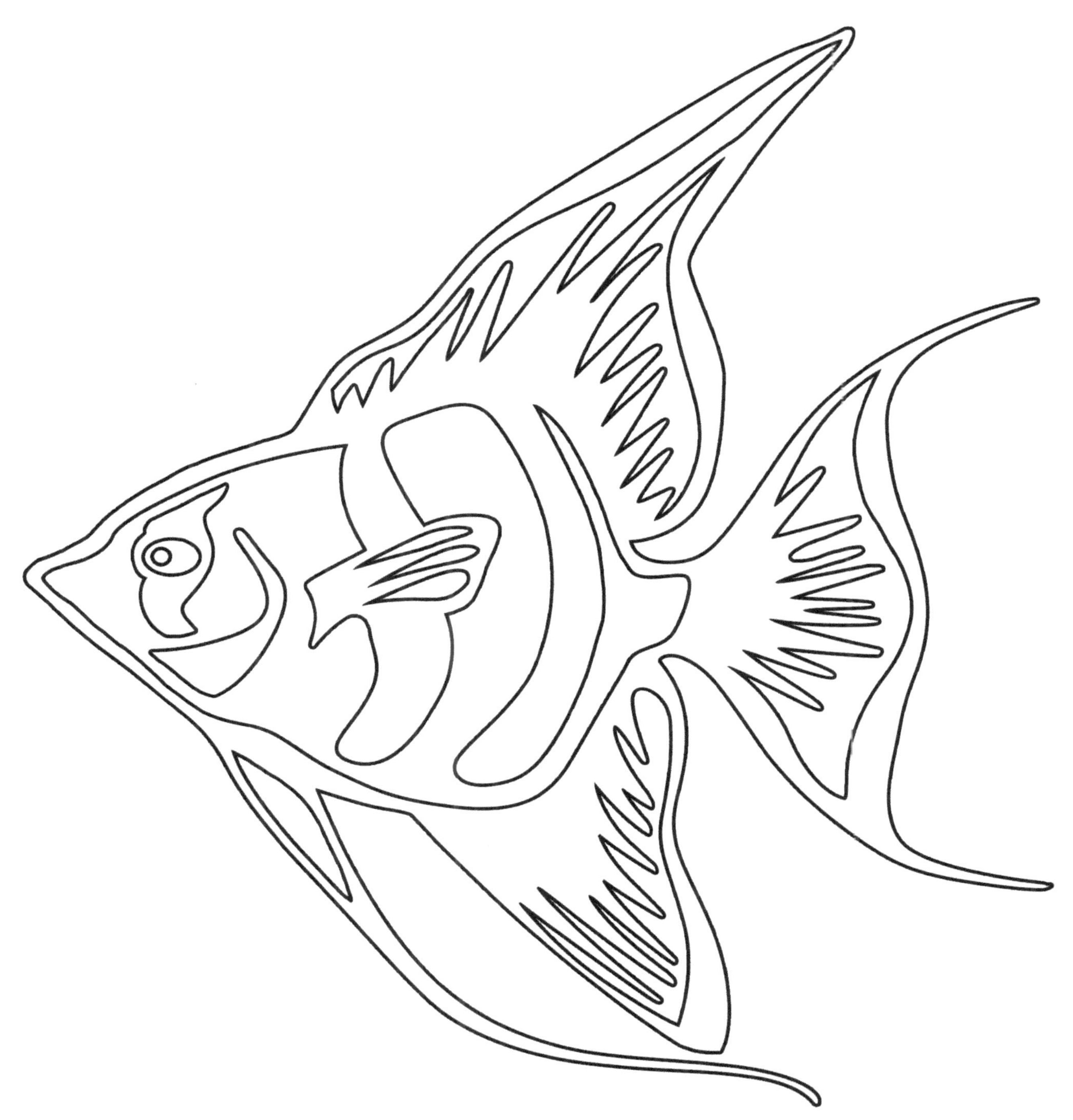

Have Faith

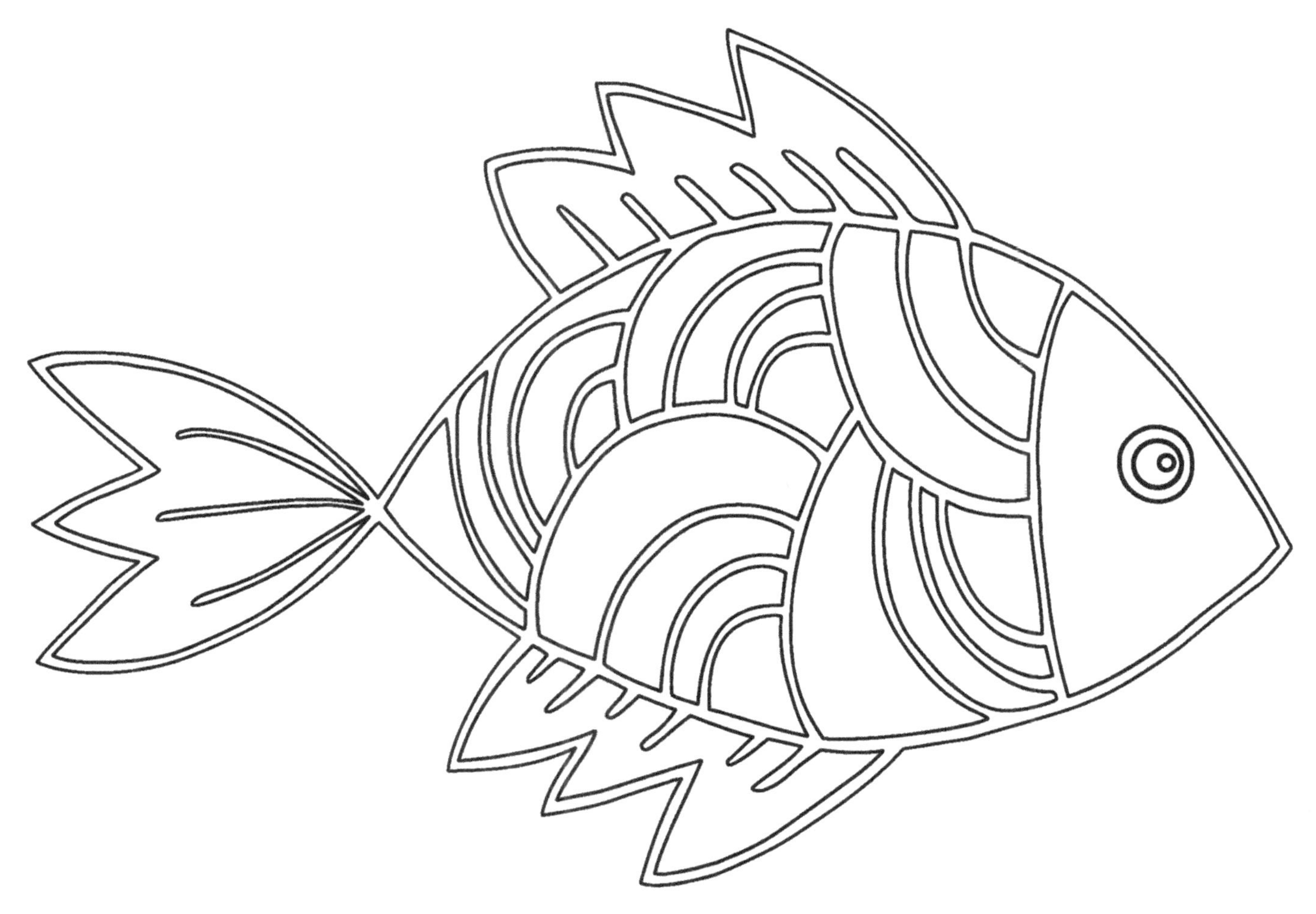

Have Patience

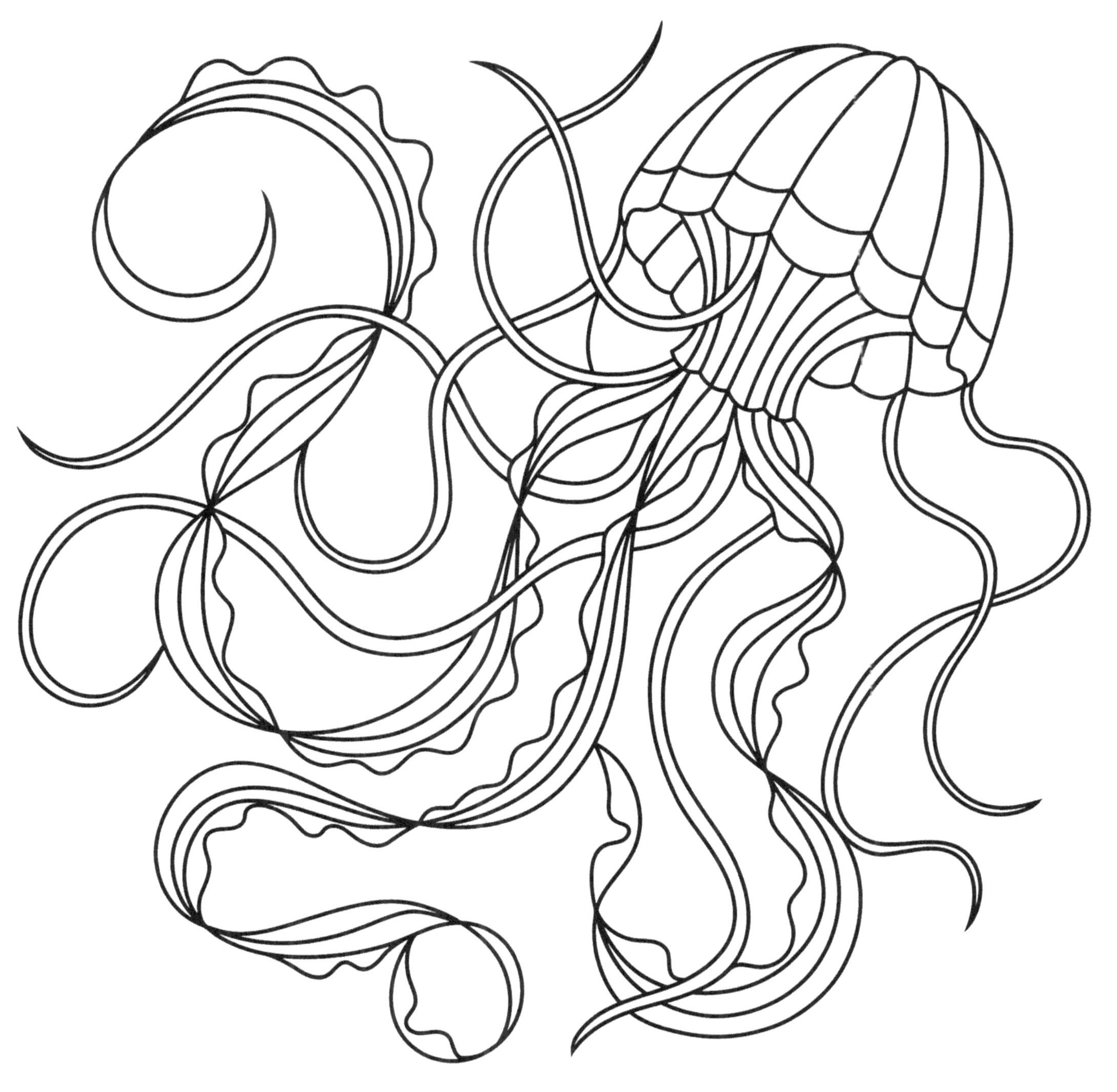

Hello Gorgeous

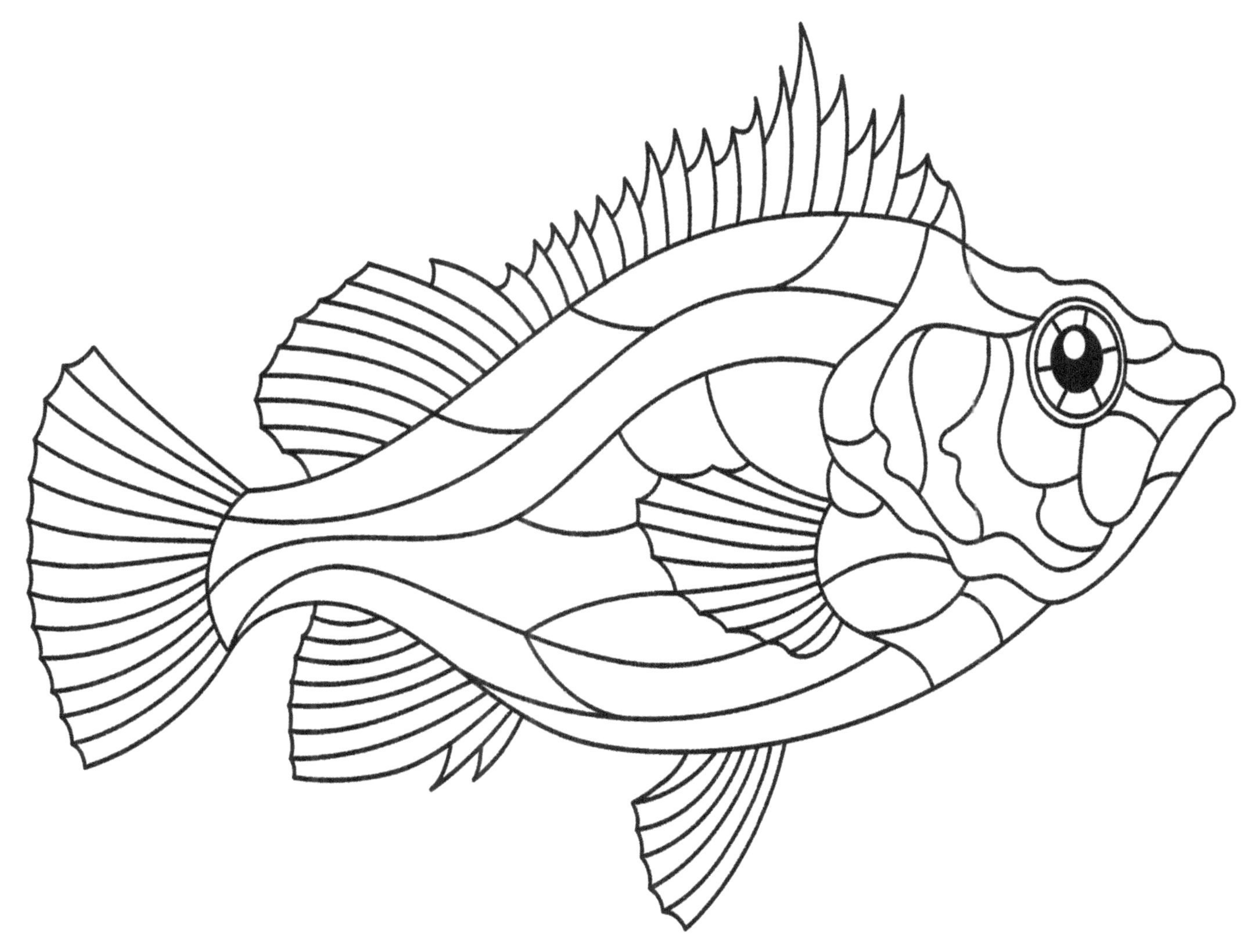

Hold On

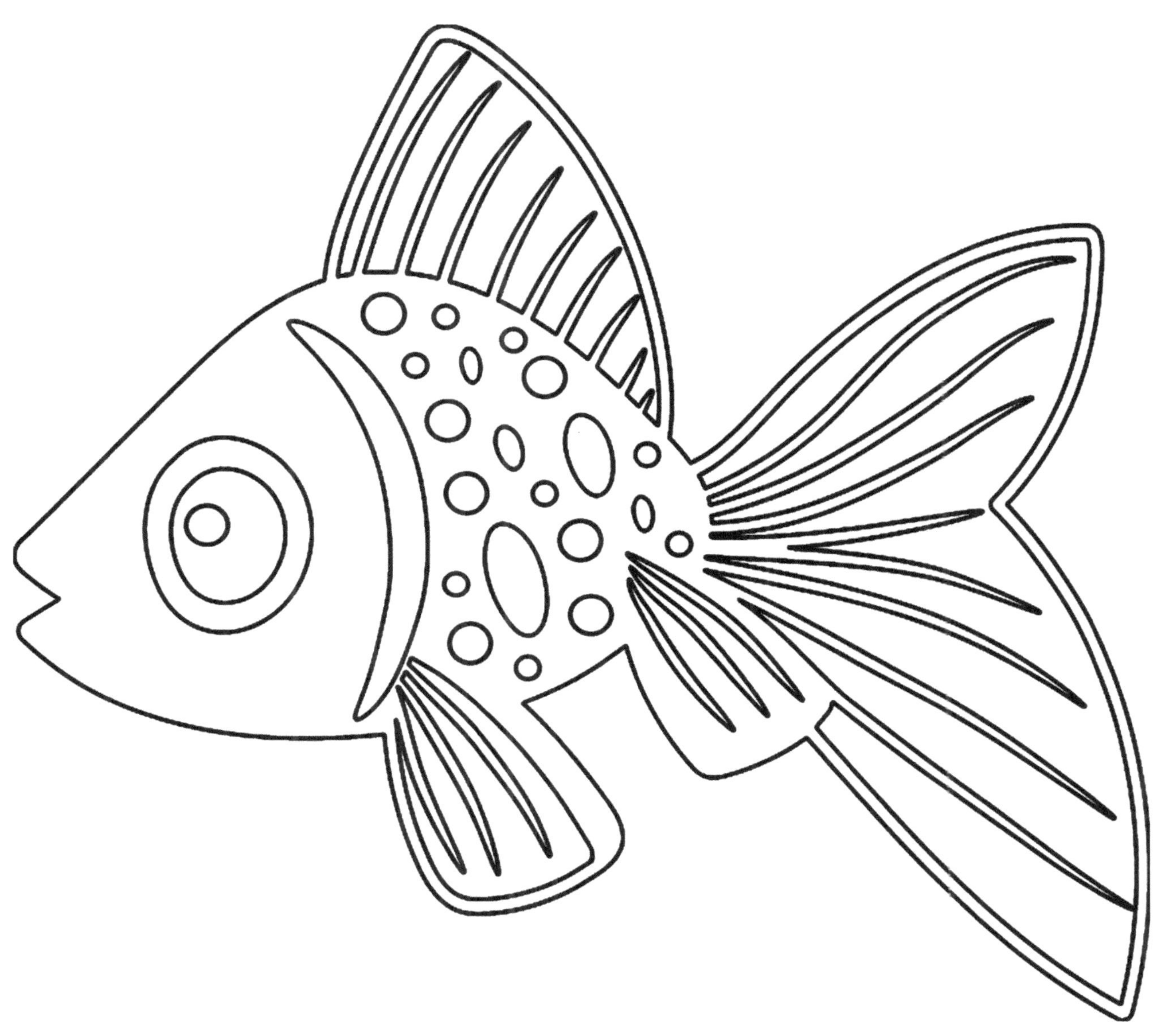

Inner Peace

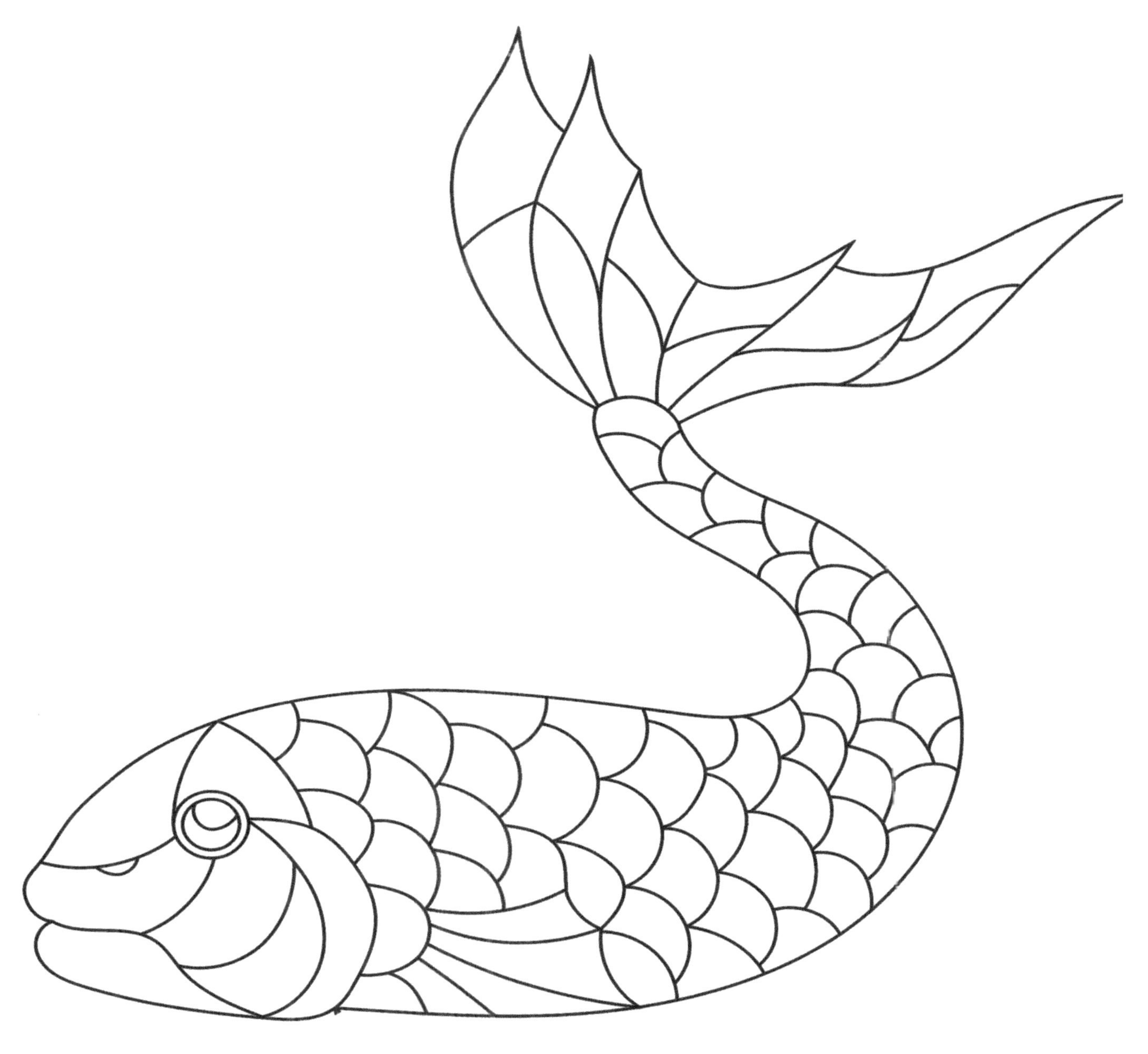

Invite Tranquility

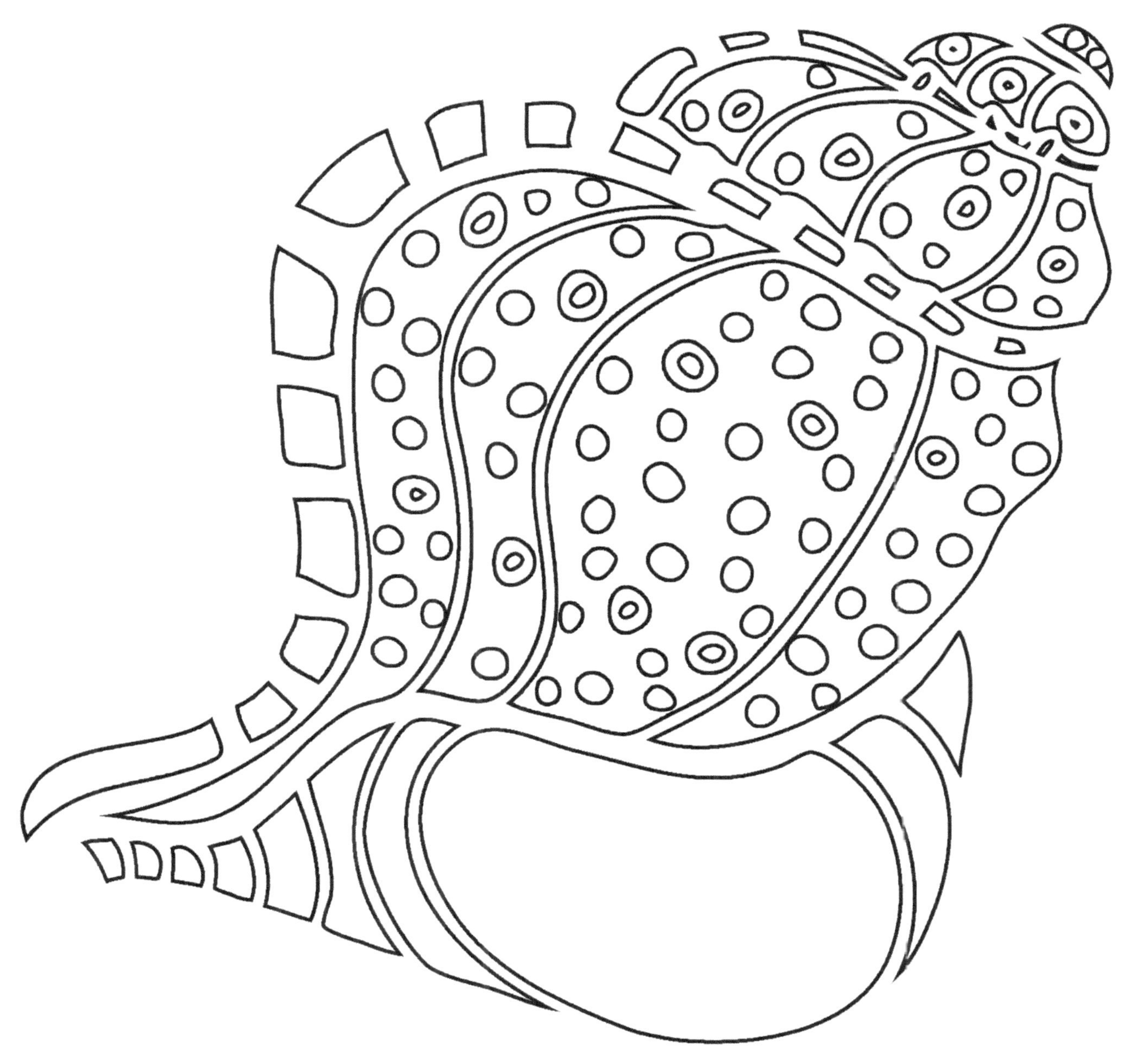

Just Believe

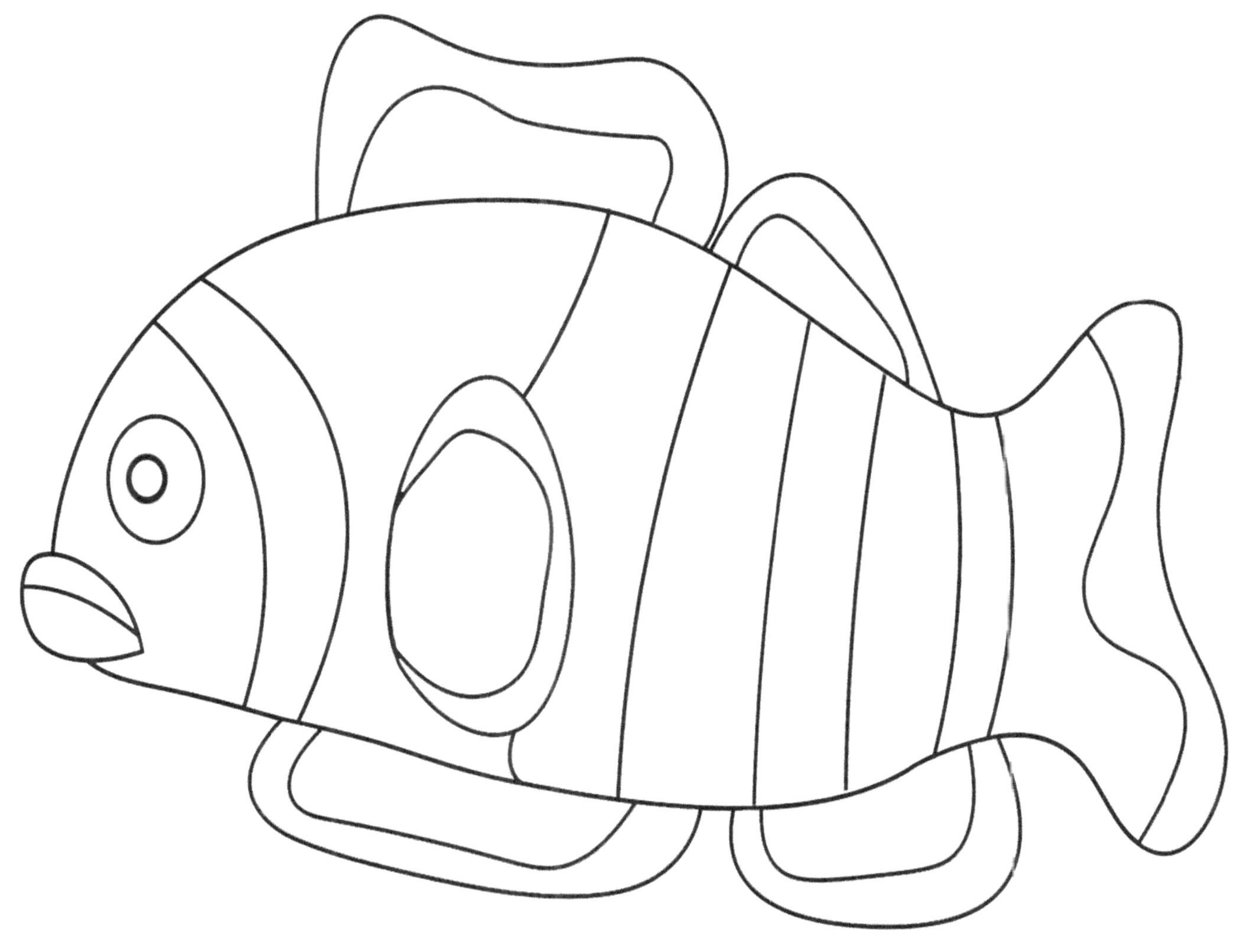

Just Breathe

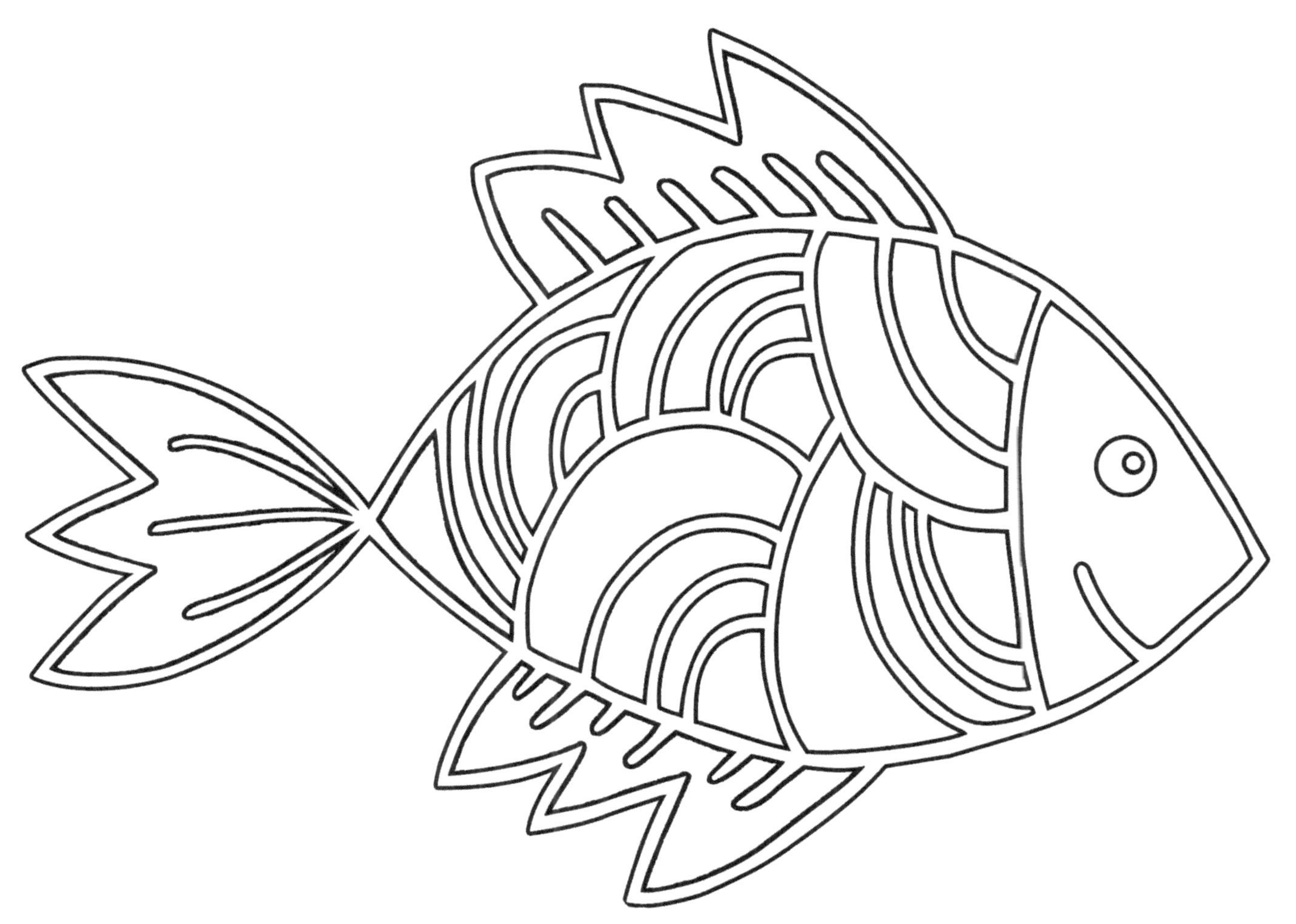

Just Imagine

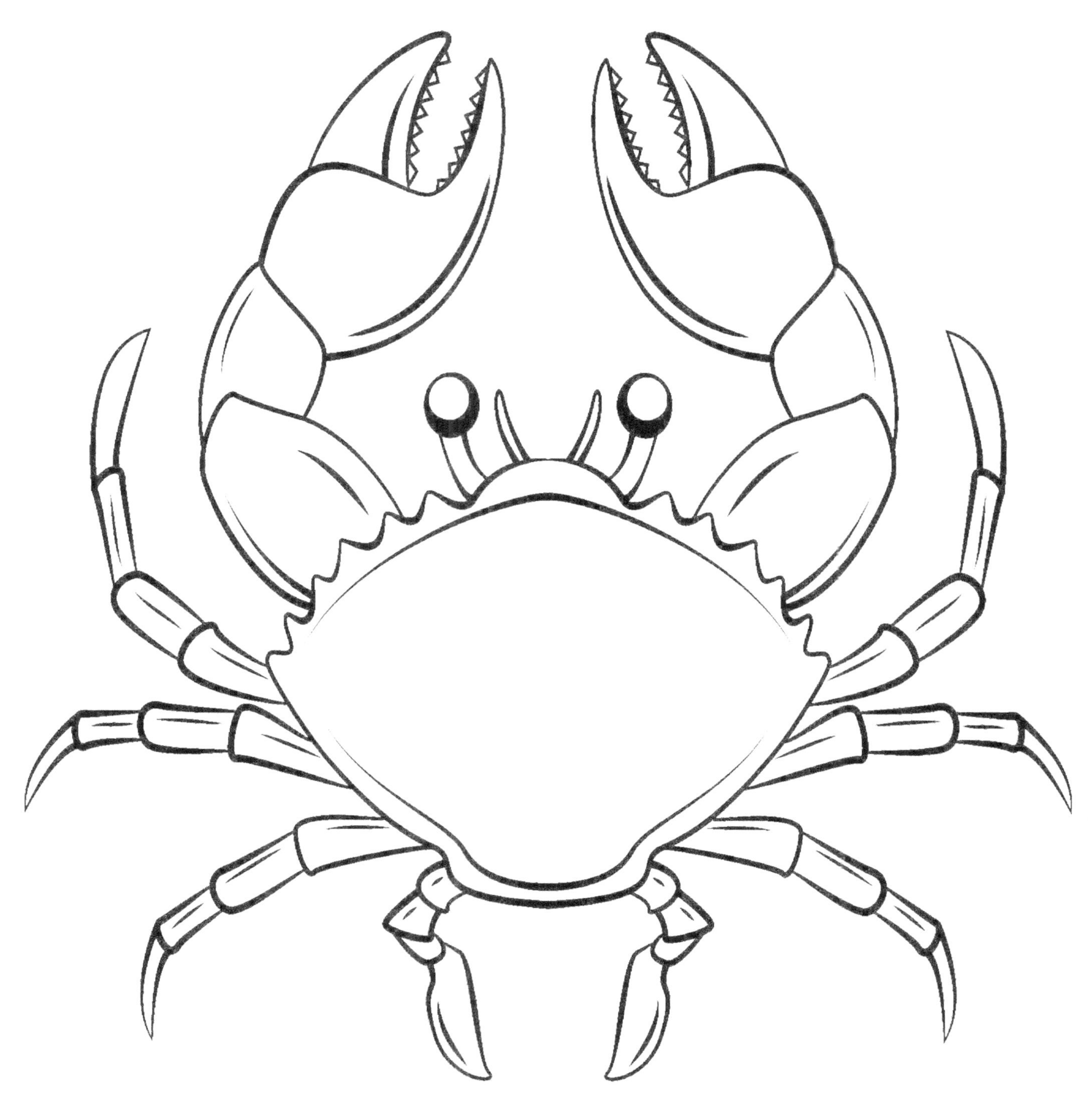

Just Peachy

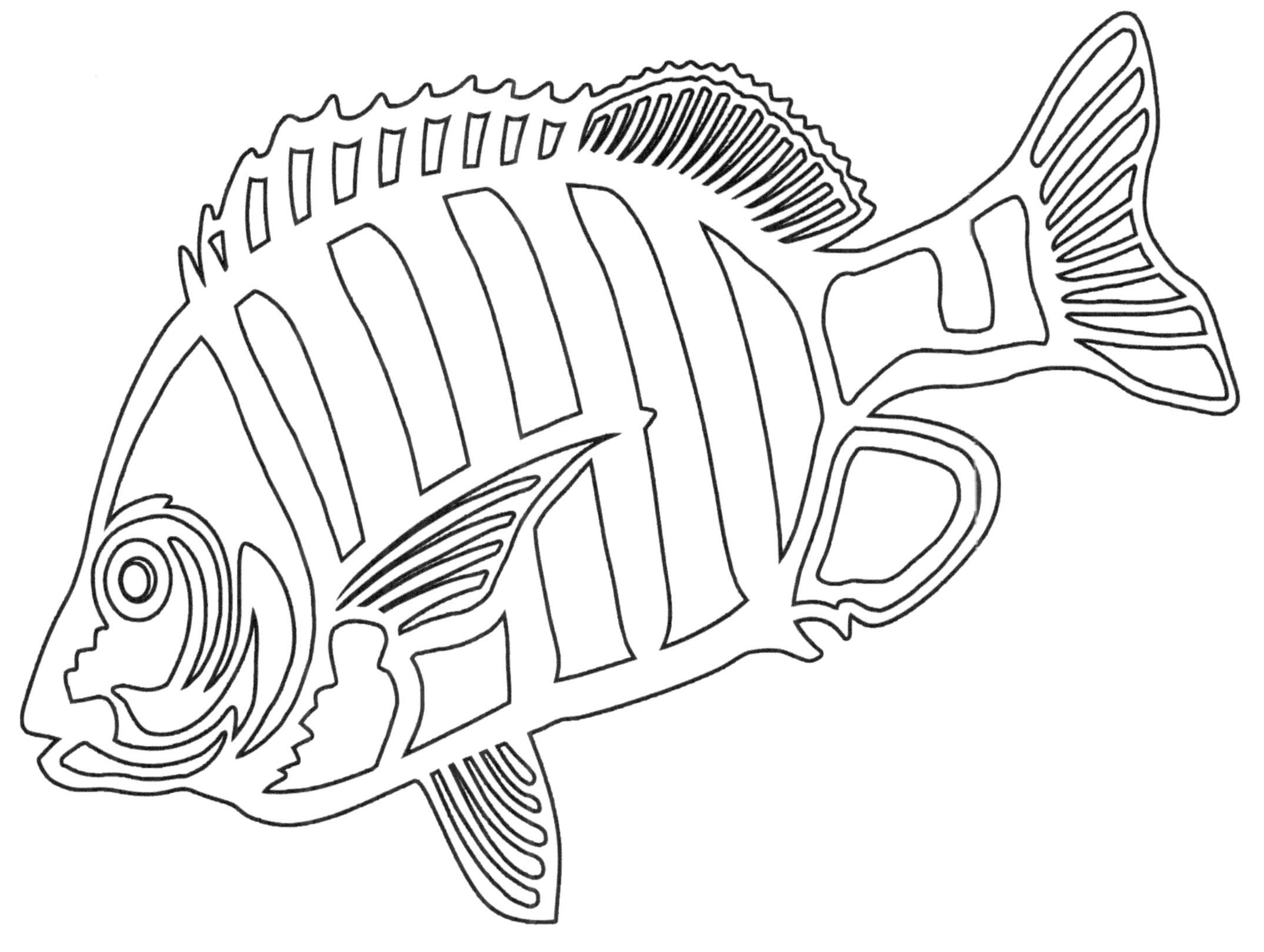

Keep Calm

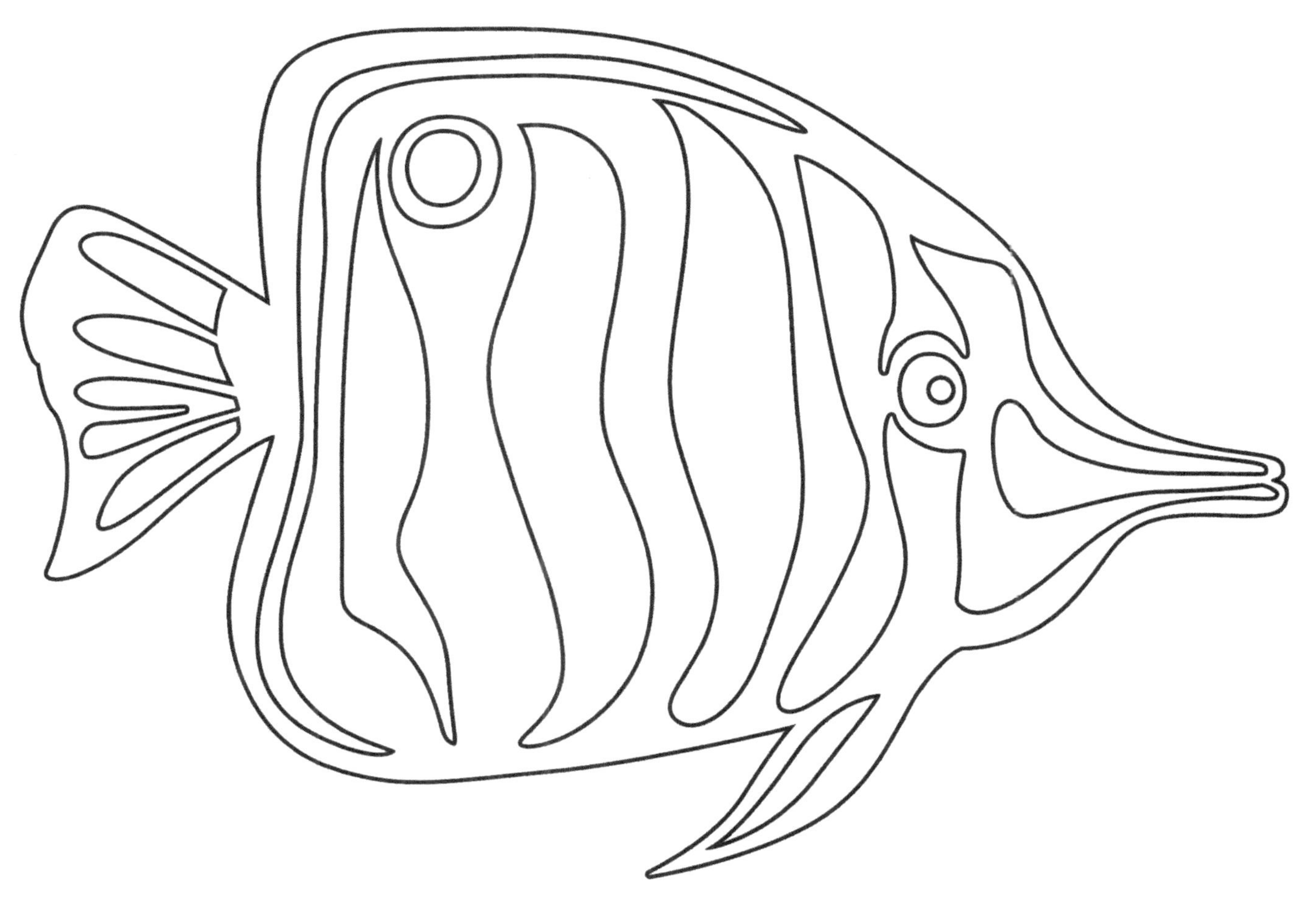

Keep Dreaming

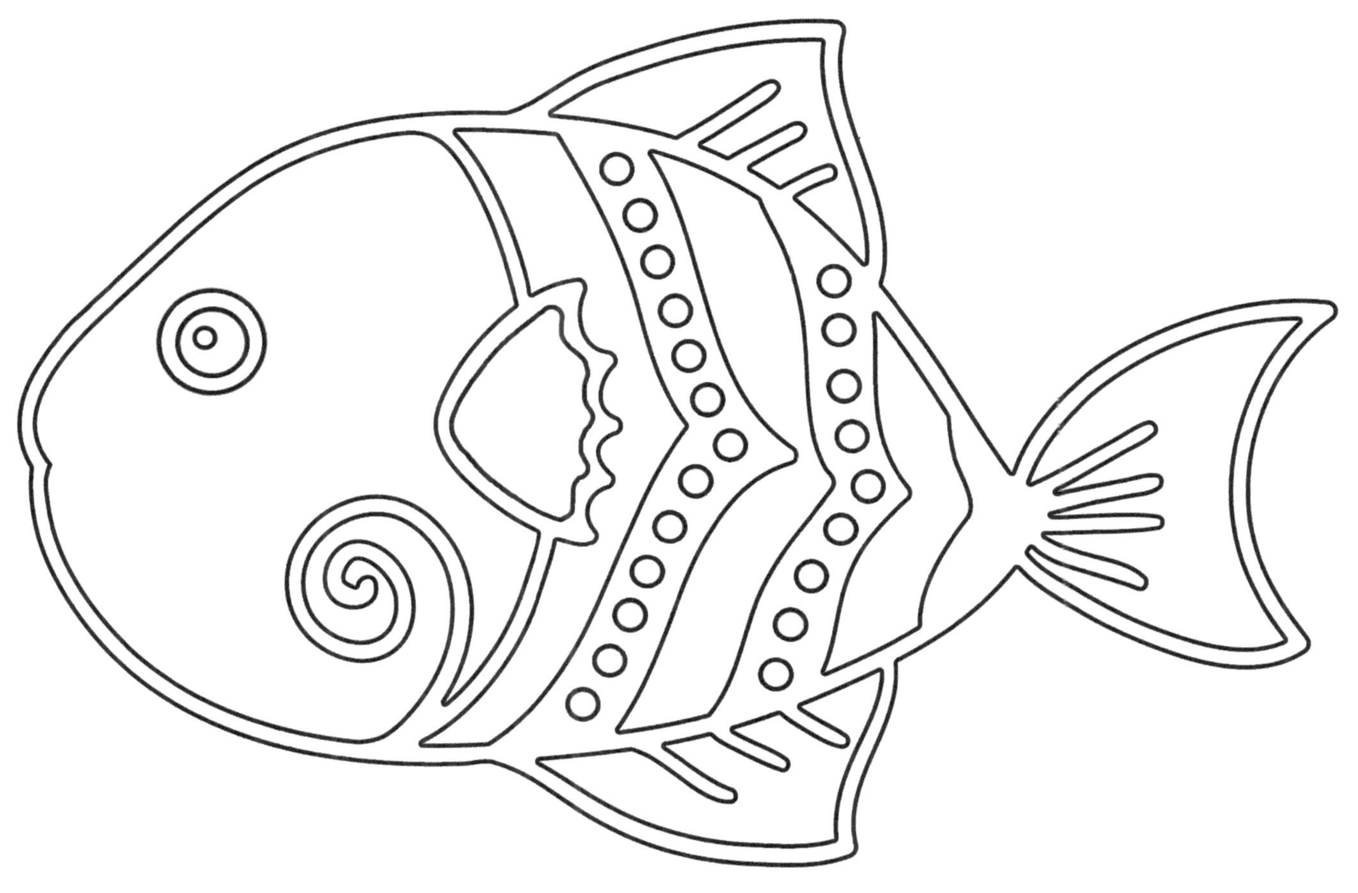

Keep Going

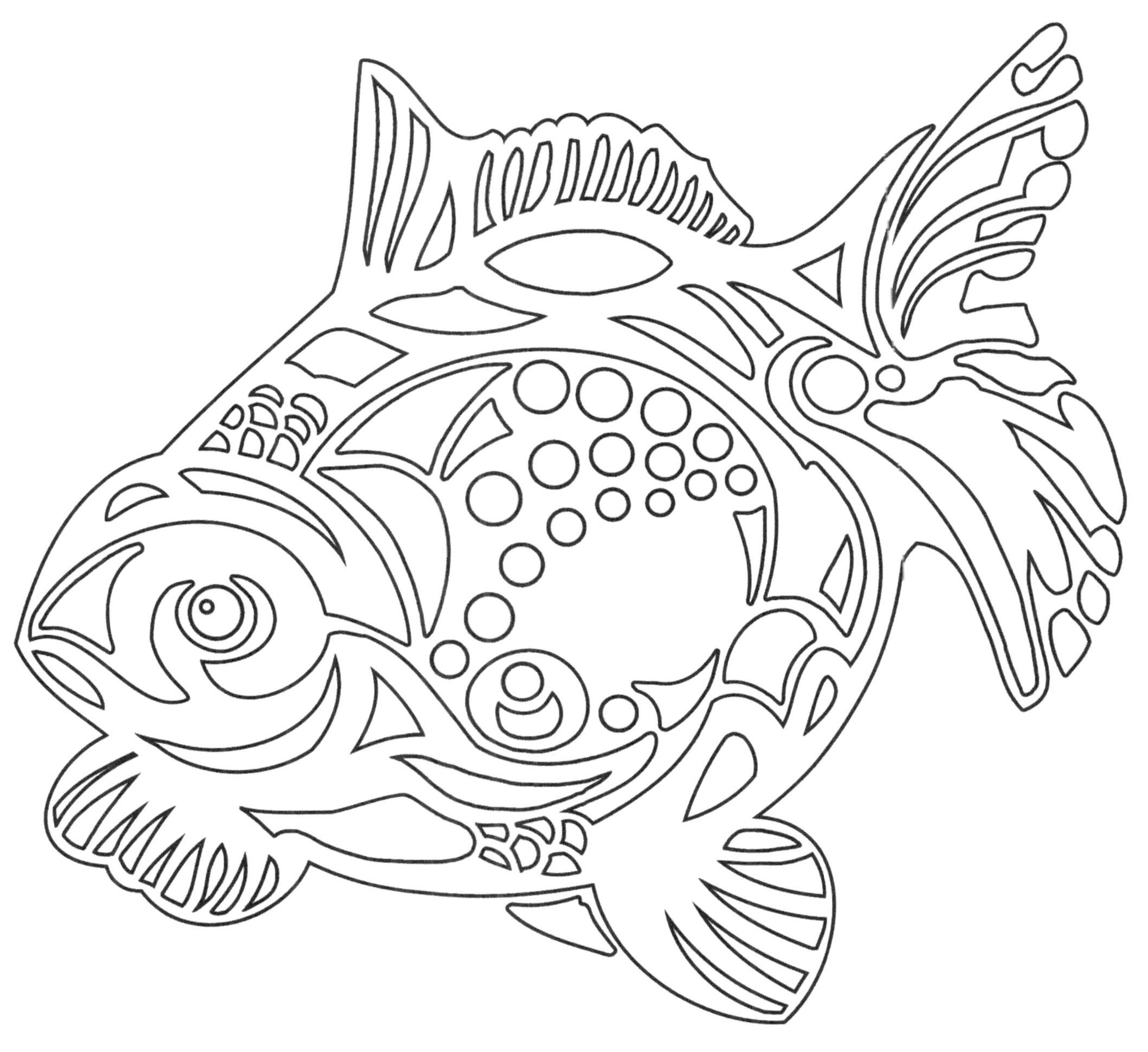

Keep Smiling

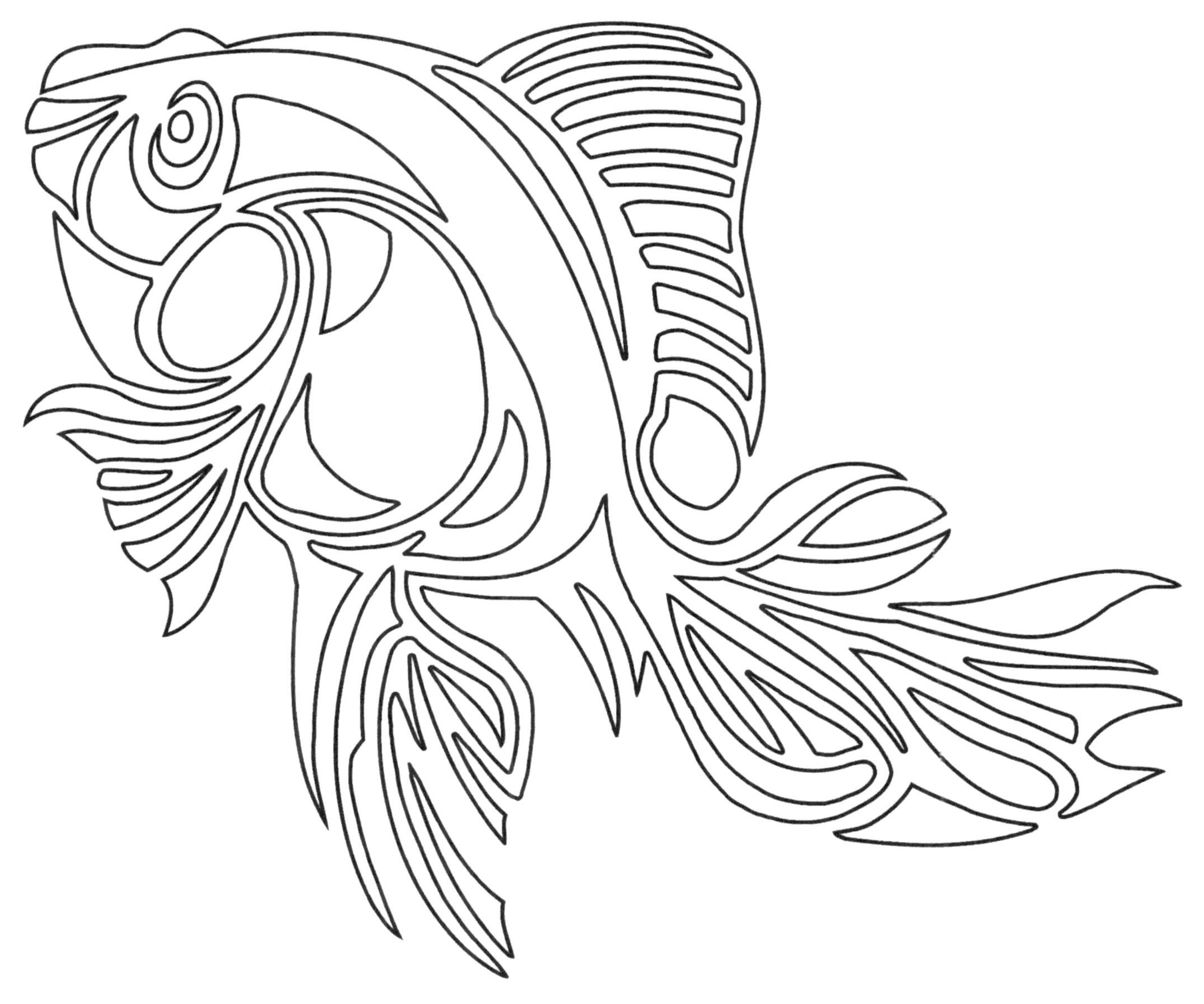

Laughter Heals

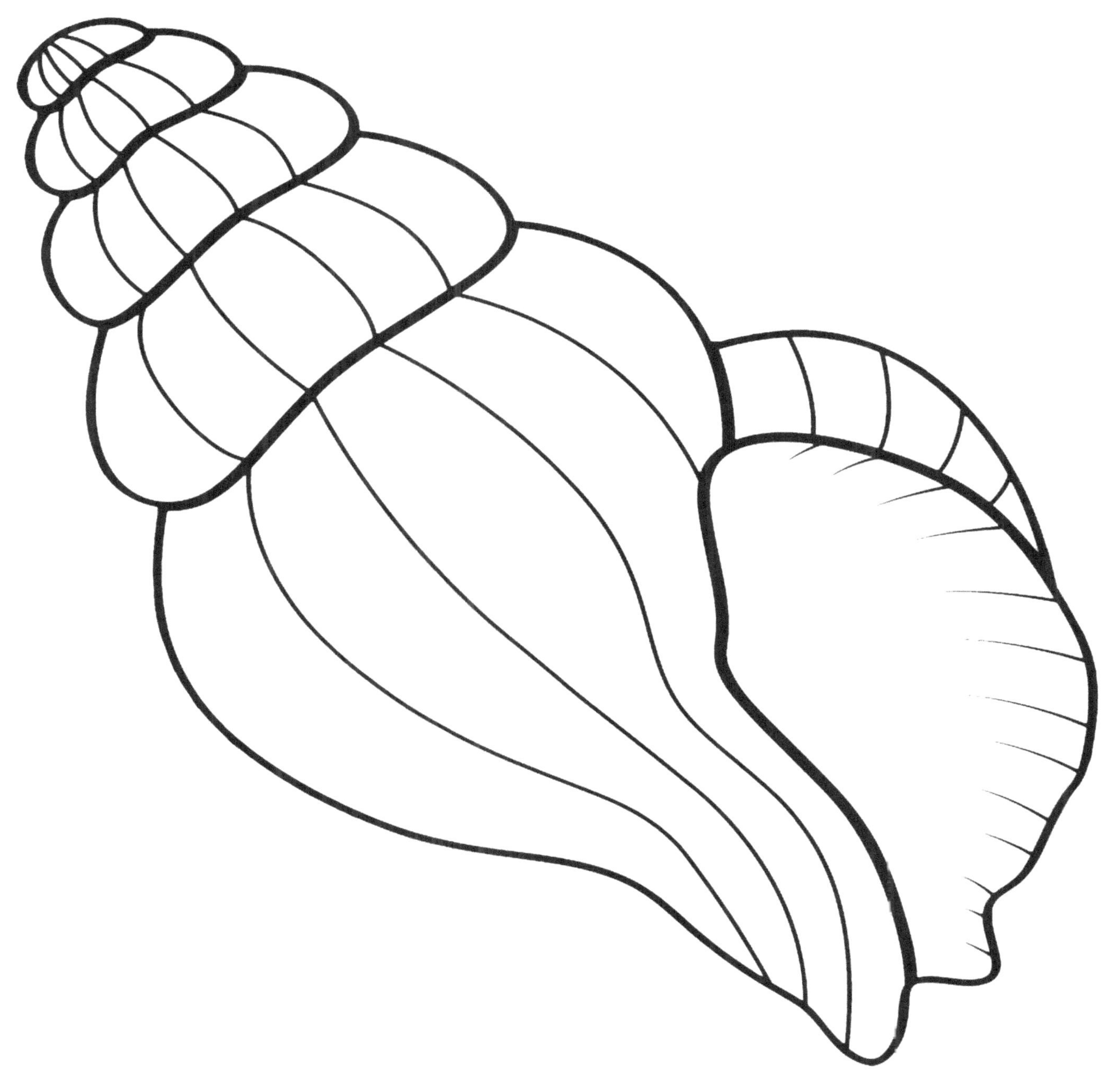

Let Go

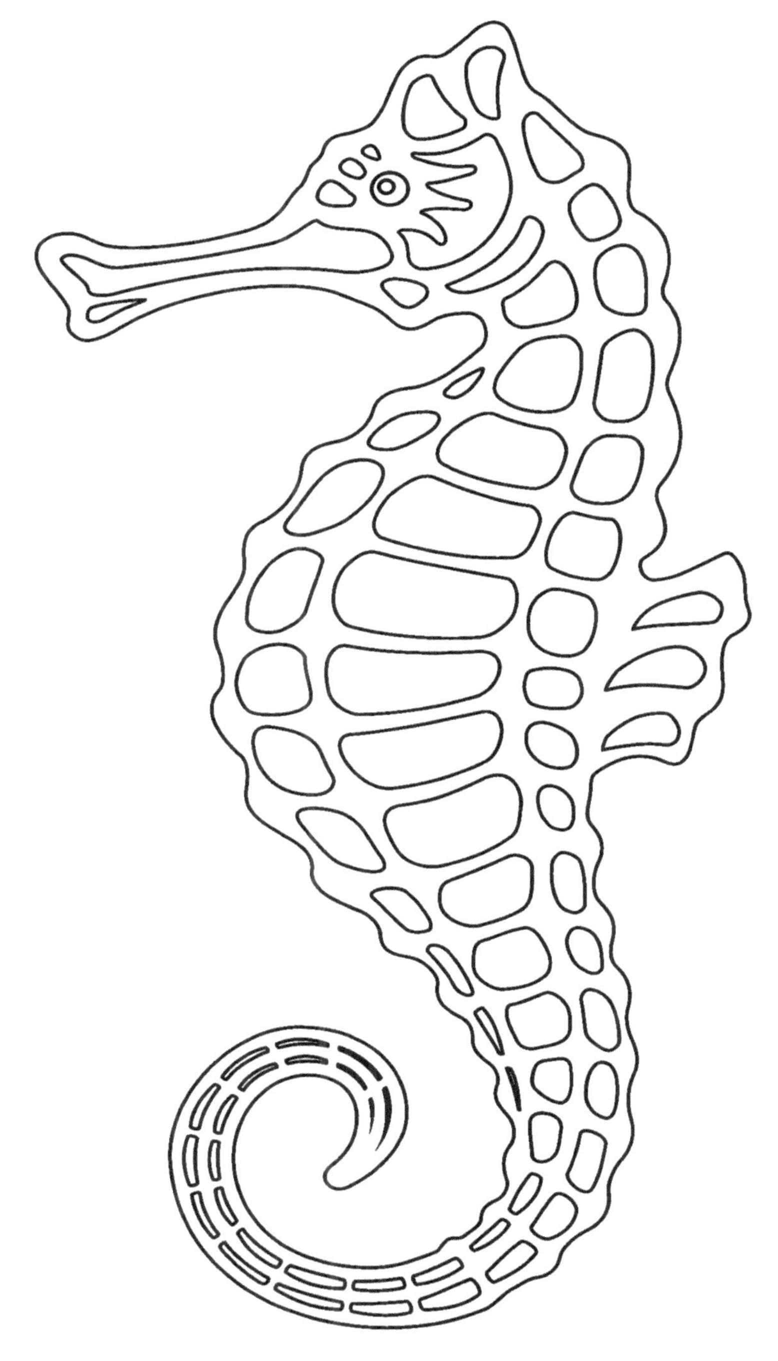

Look Within

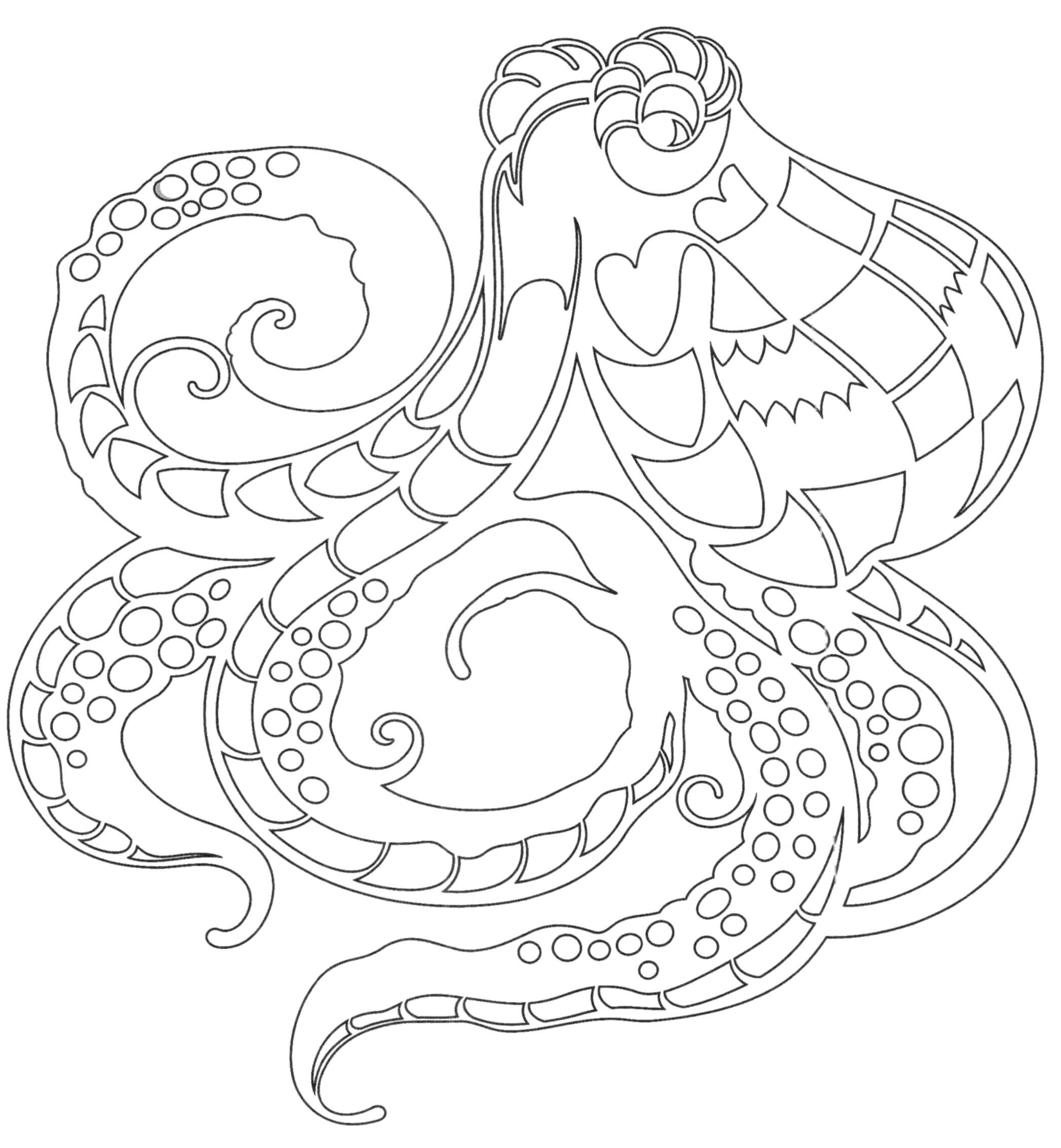

Loosen Up

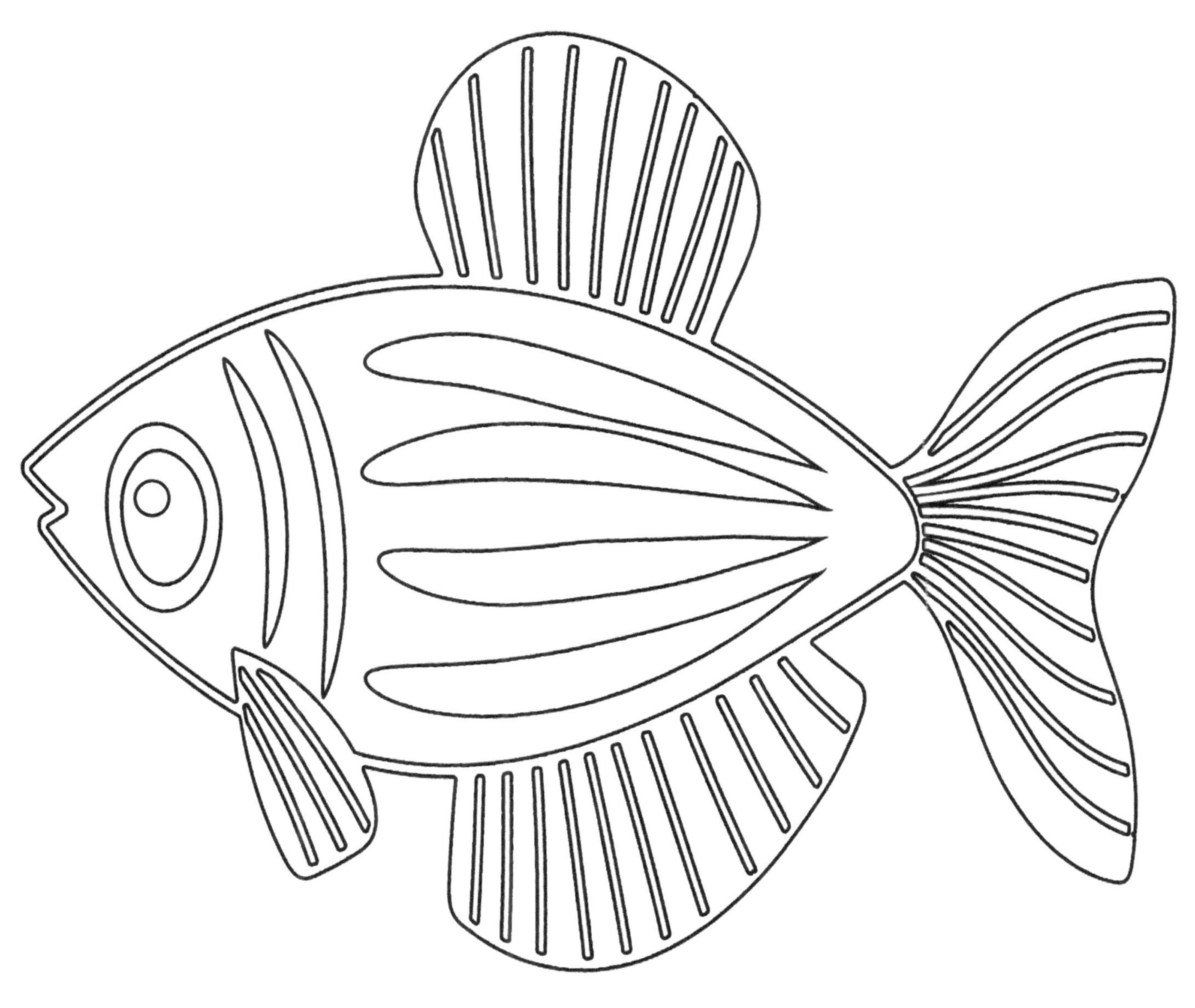

Love Endures

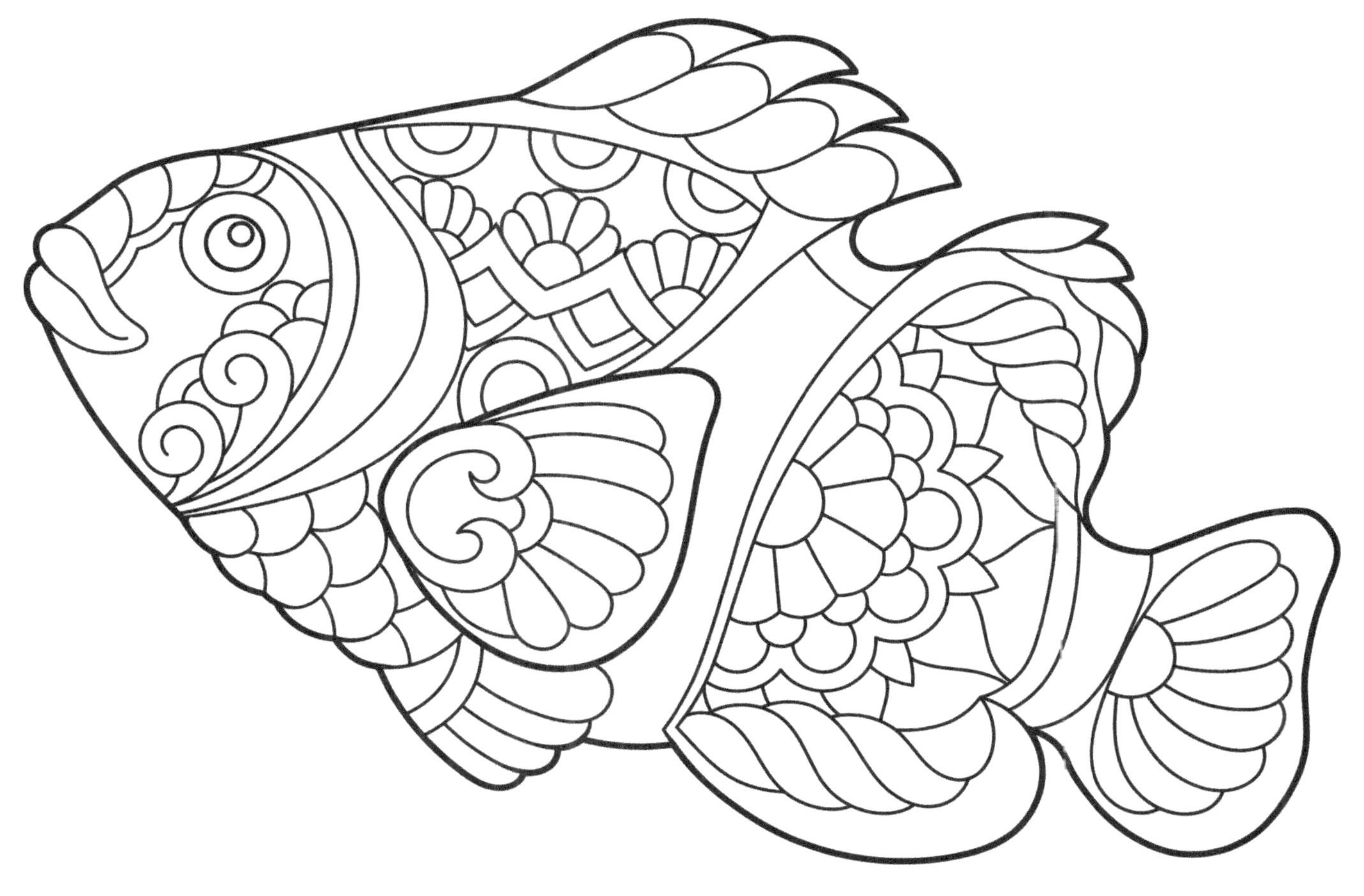

Love Heals

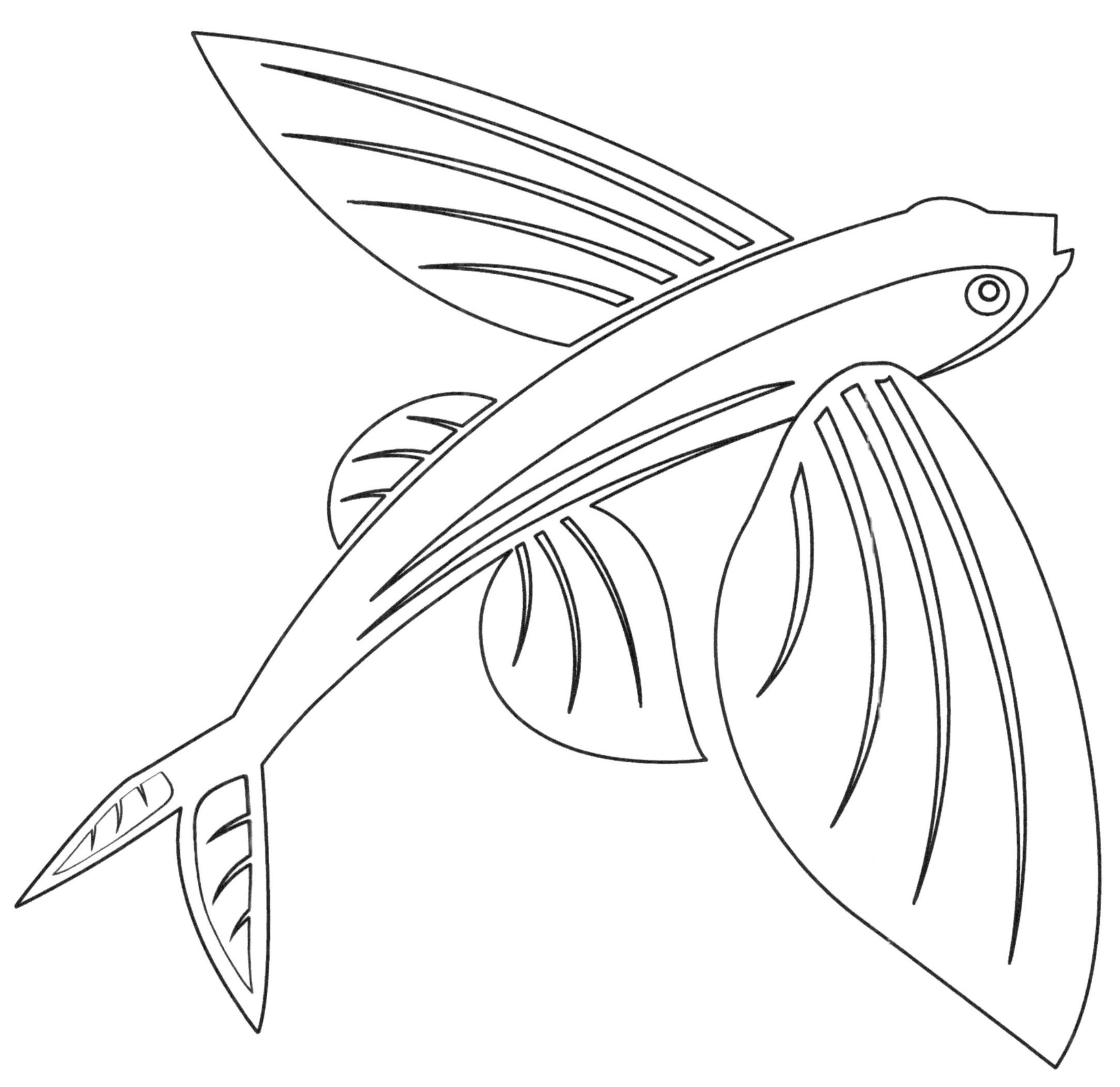

Love Life

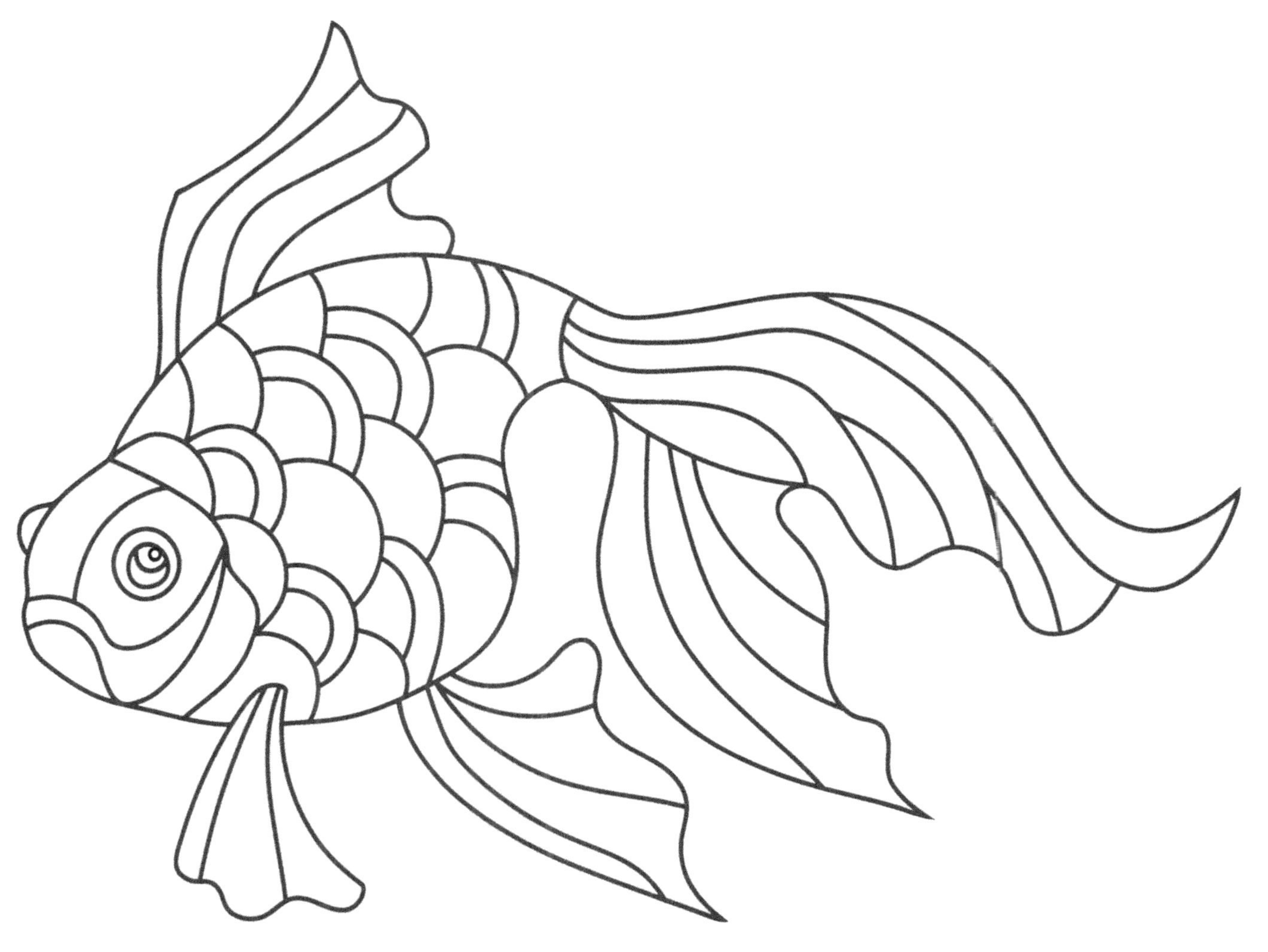

Love Yourself

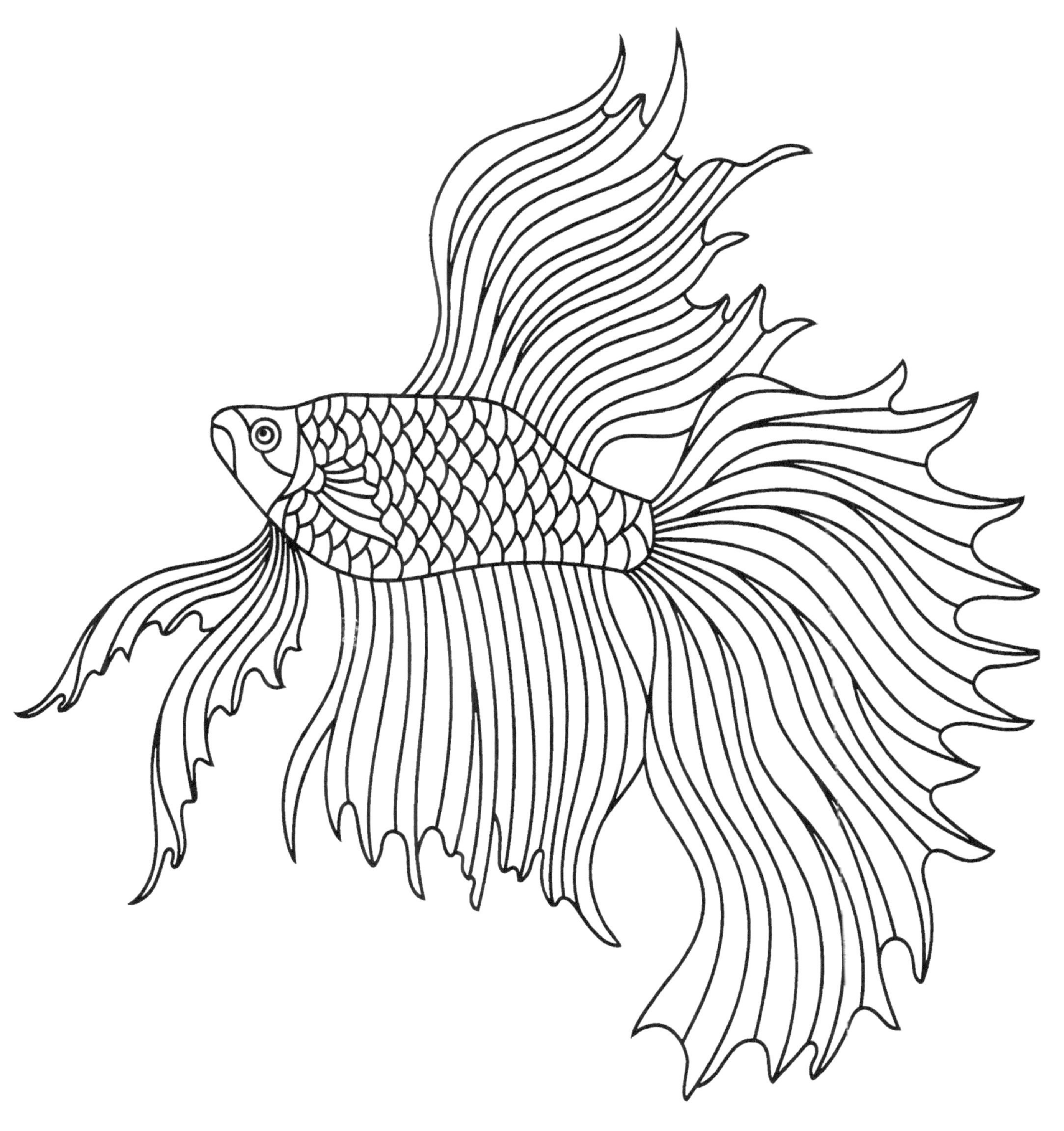

Miracles Happen

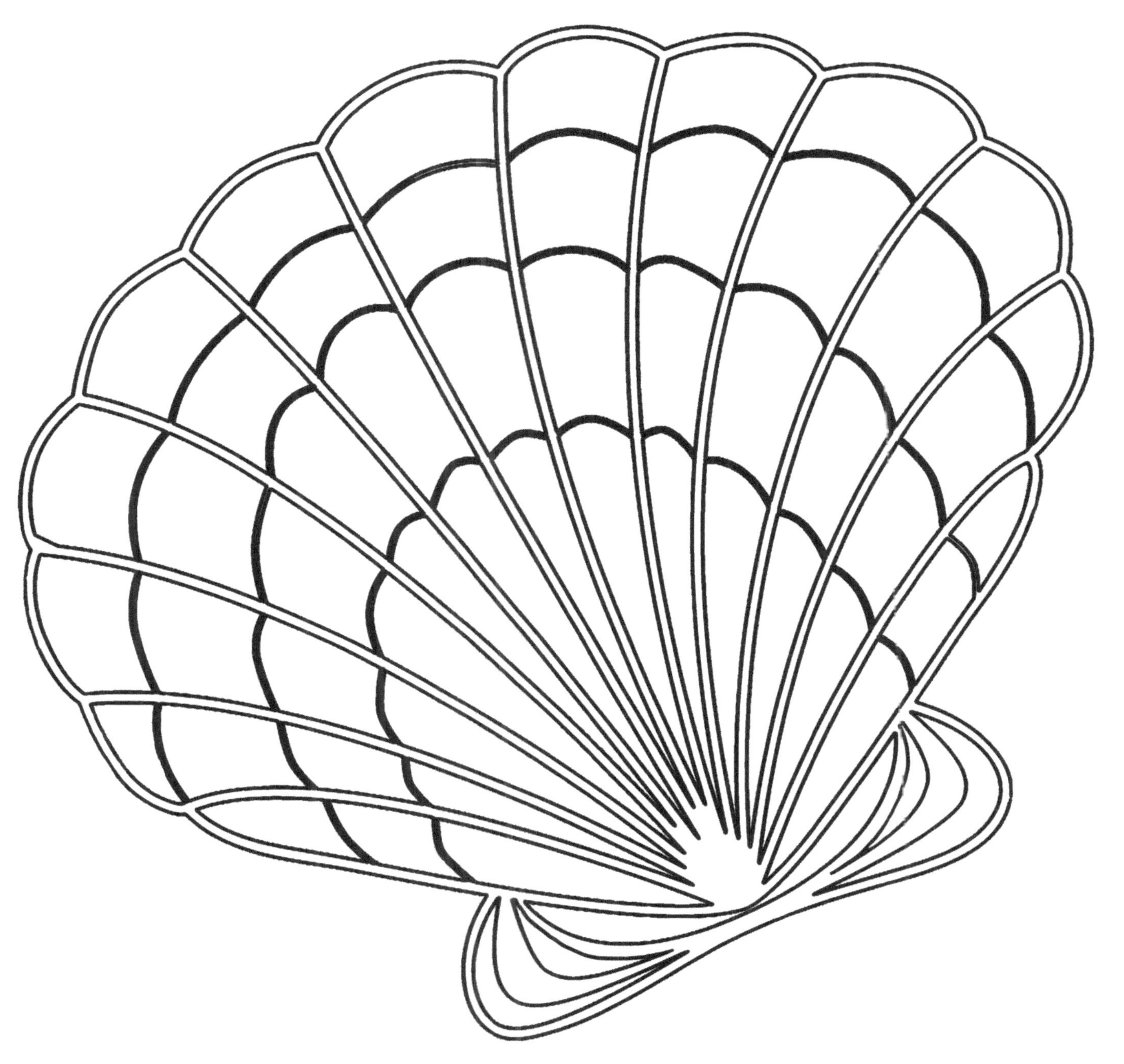

Rise Above

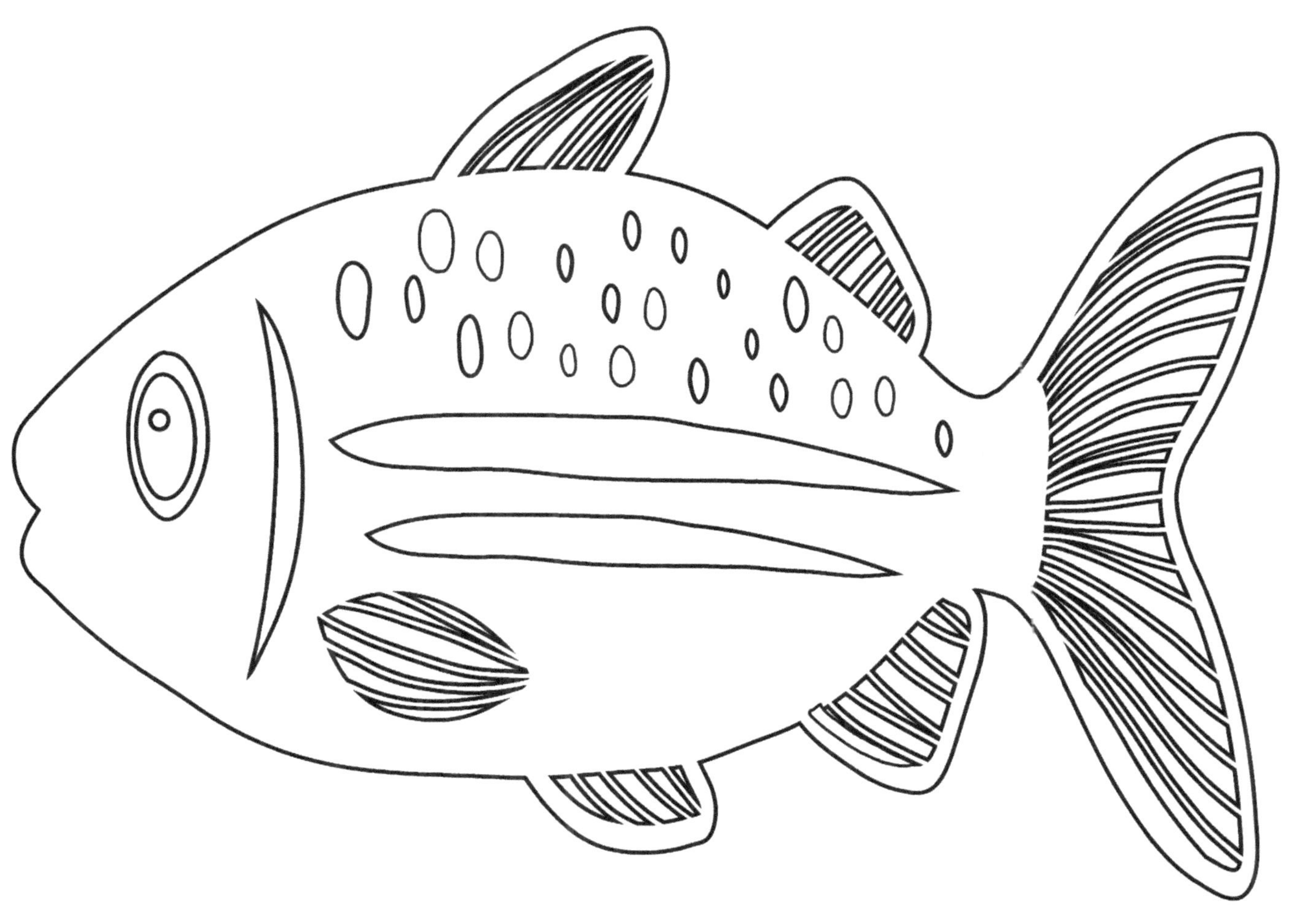

Stay Positive

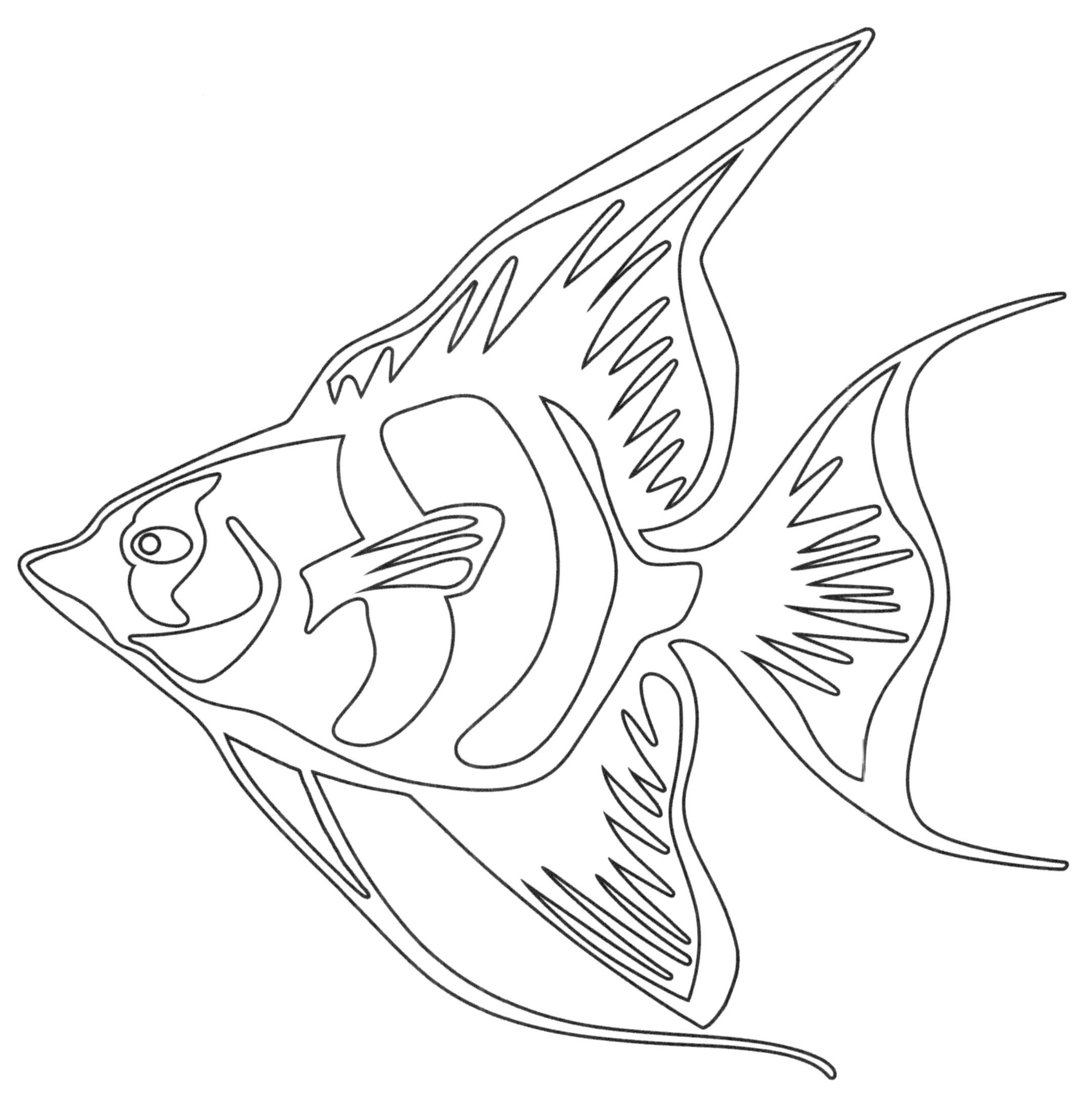

Stay Strong

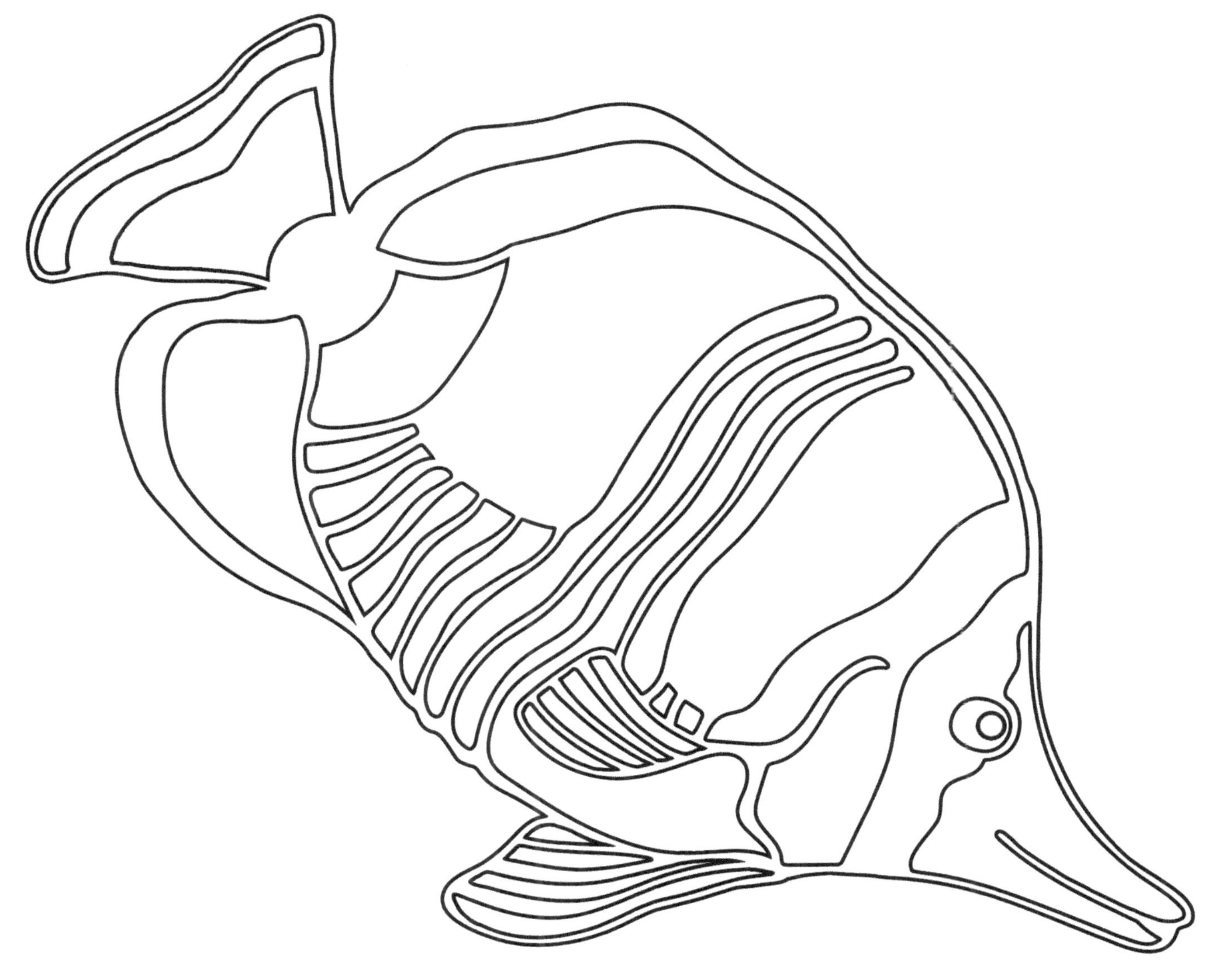

Stay True

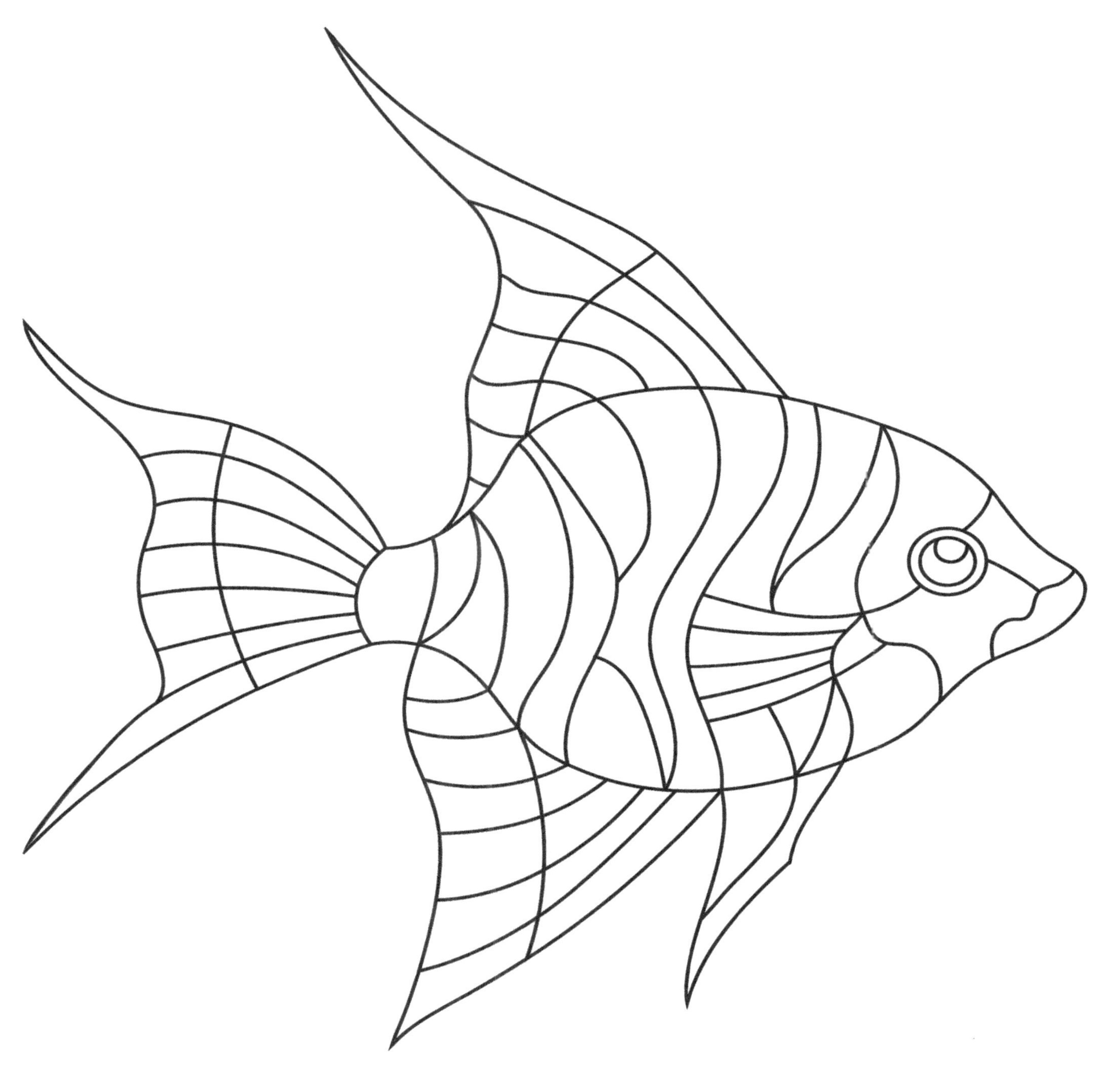

Take Care

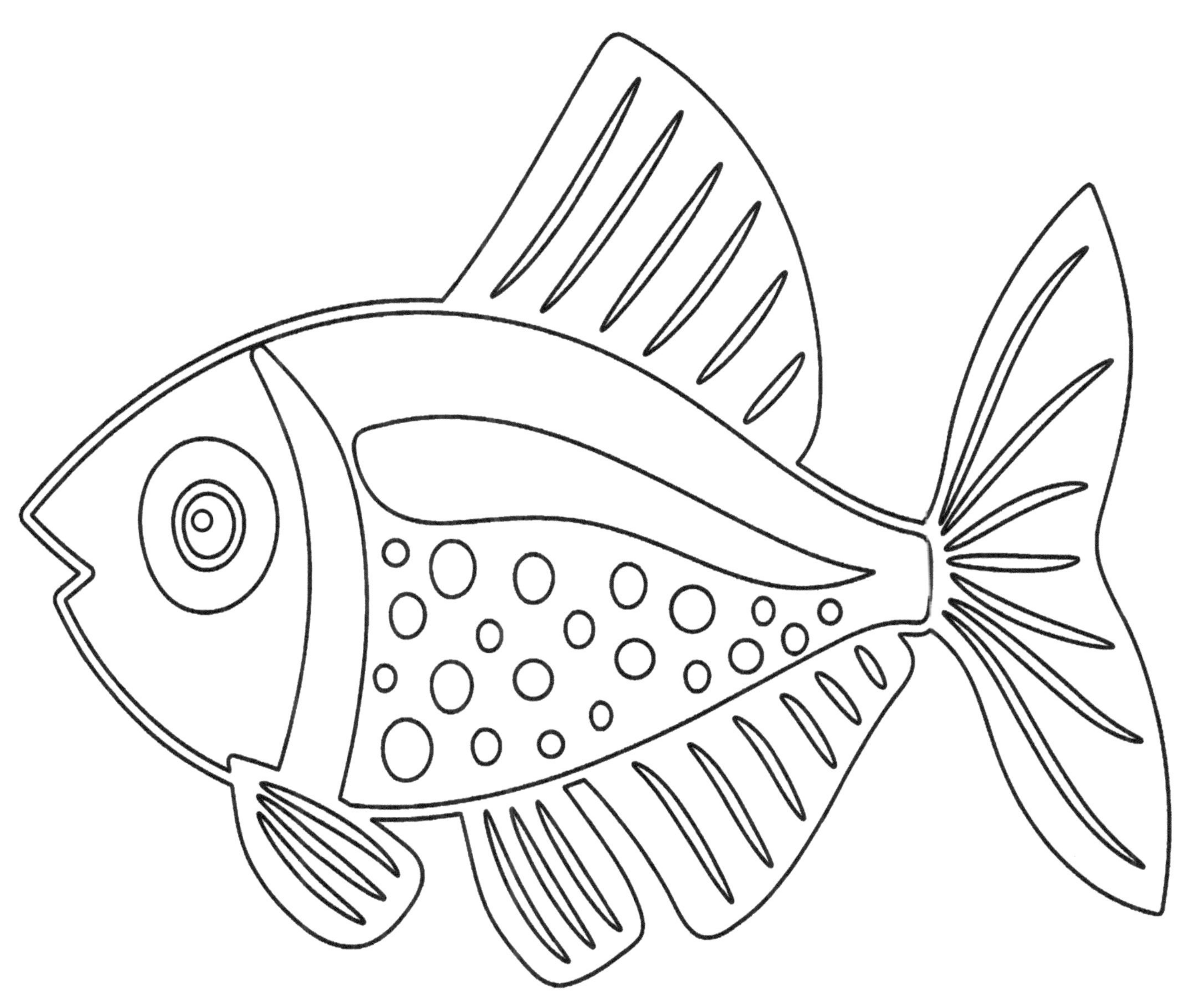

Thank You

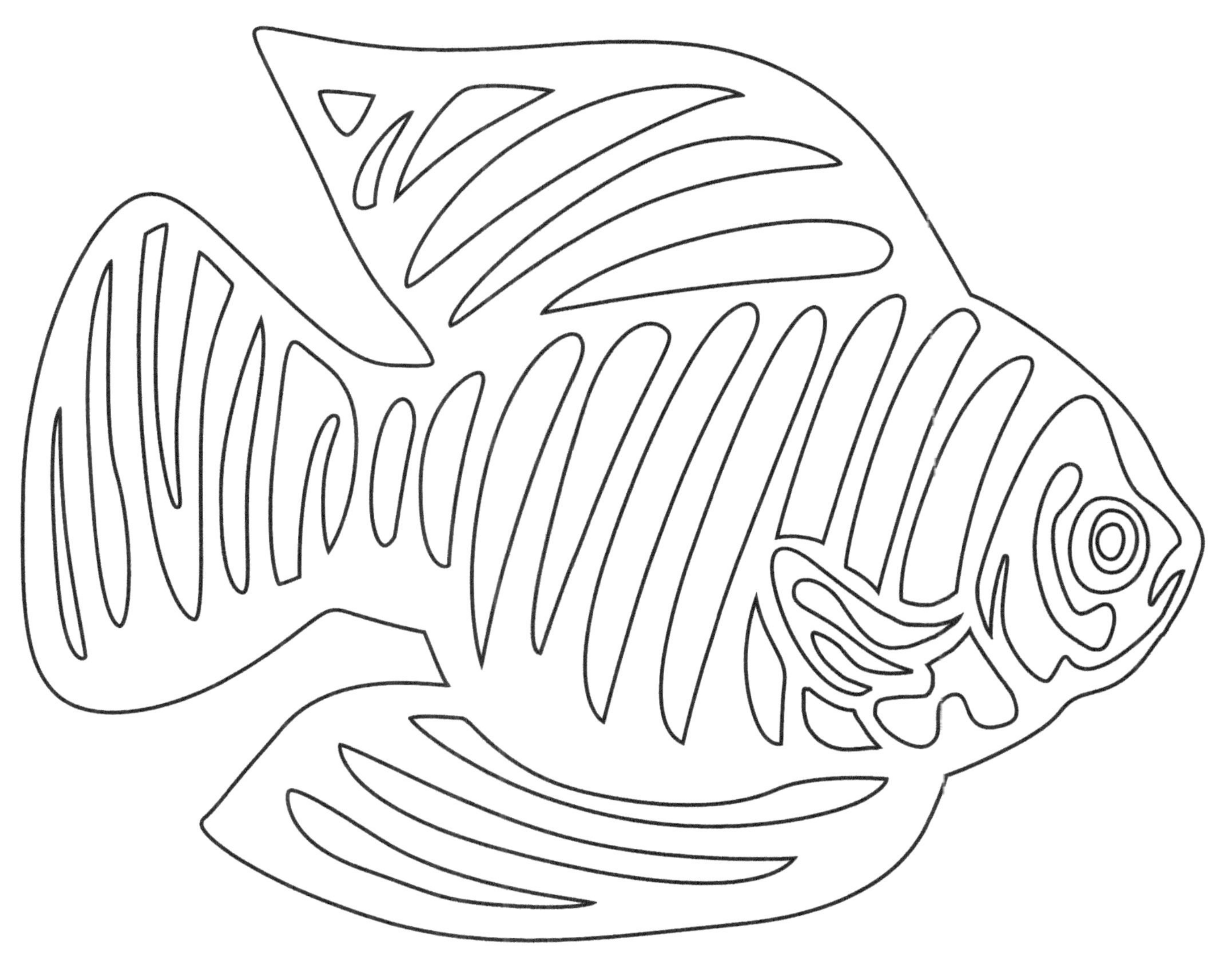

Tickled Pink

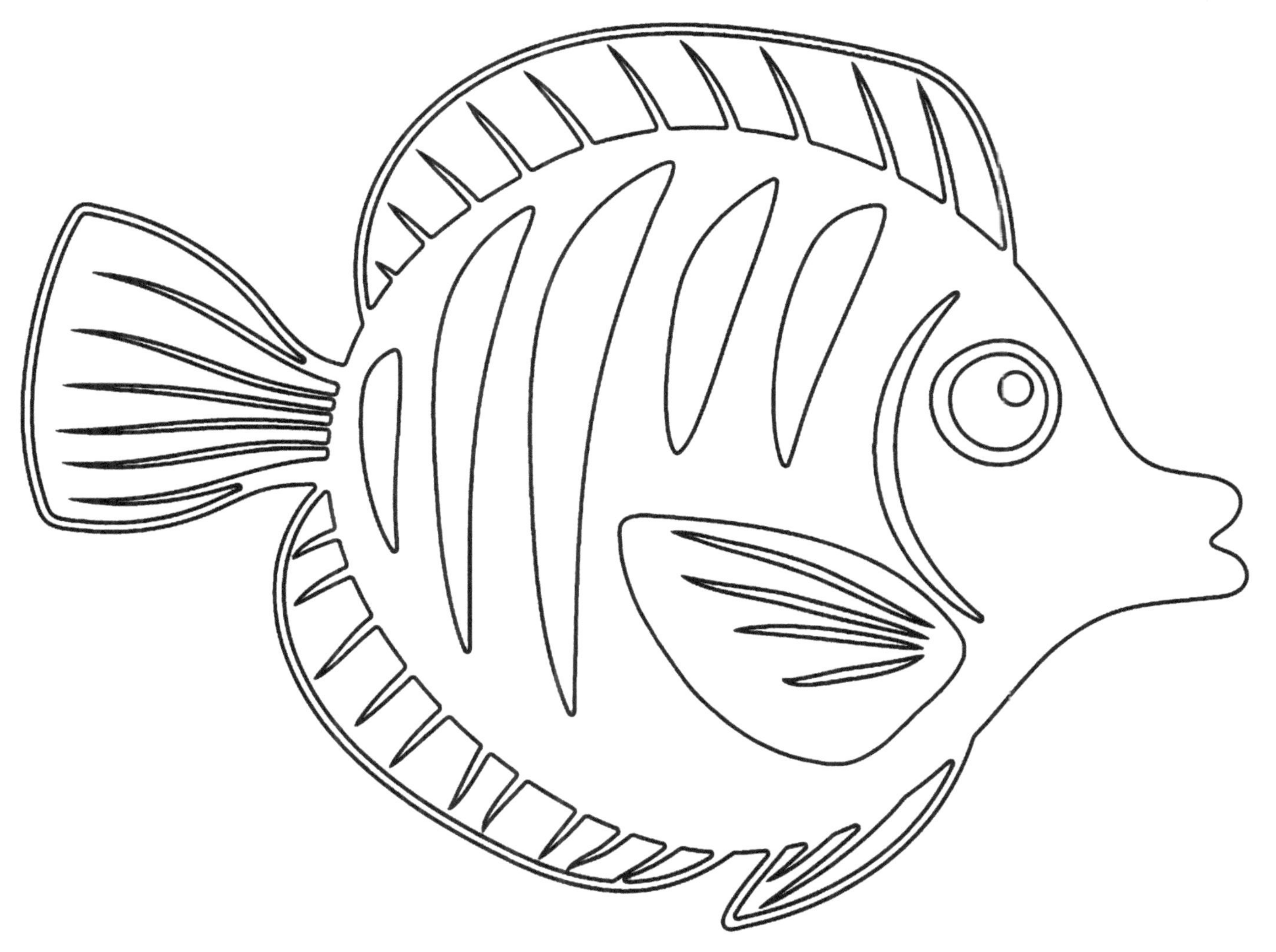

Treasure Today

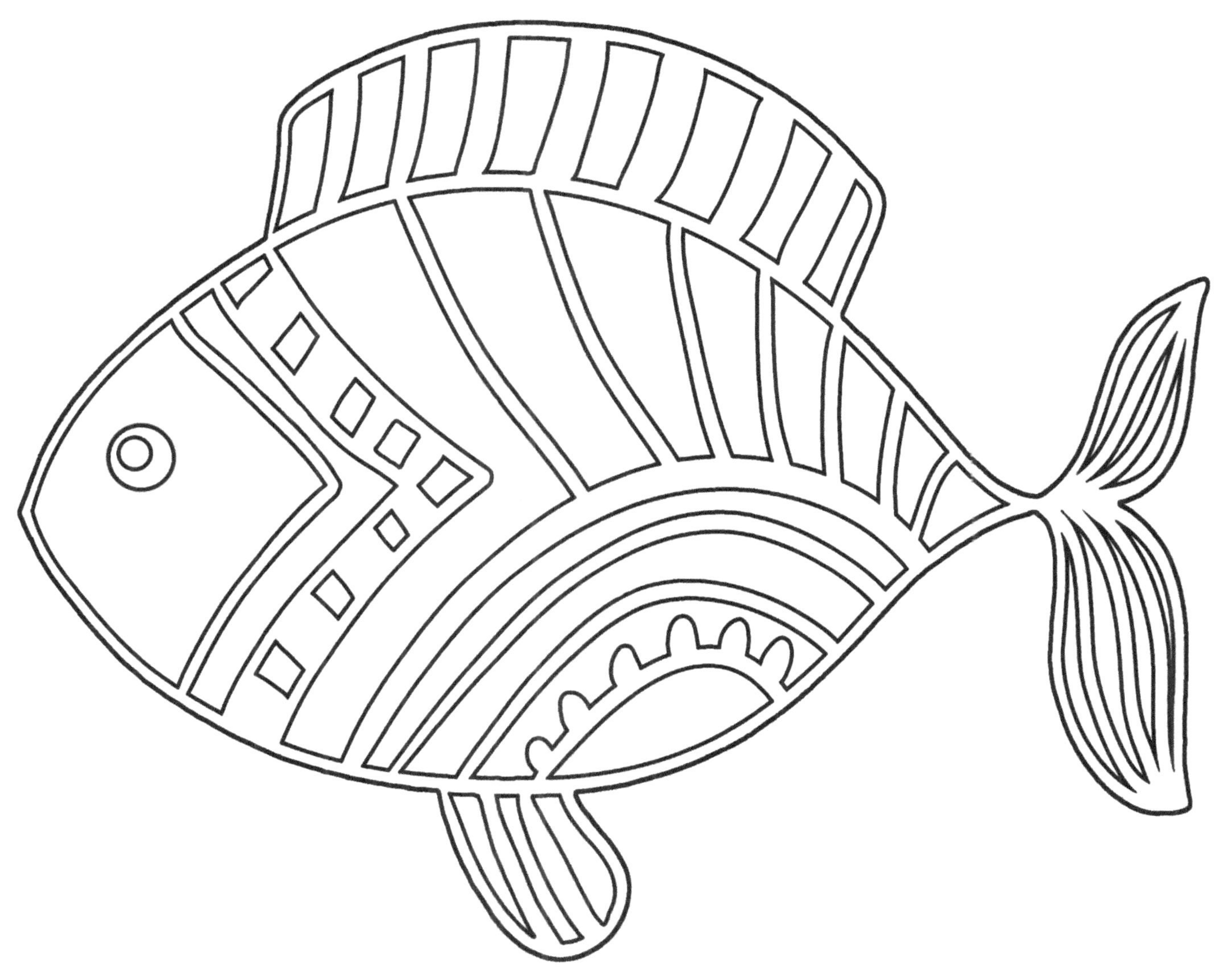

True Love

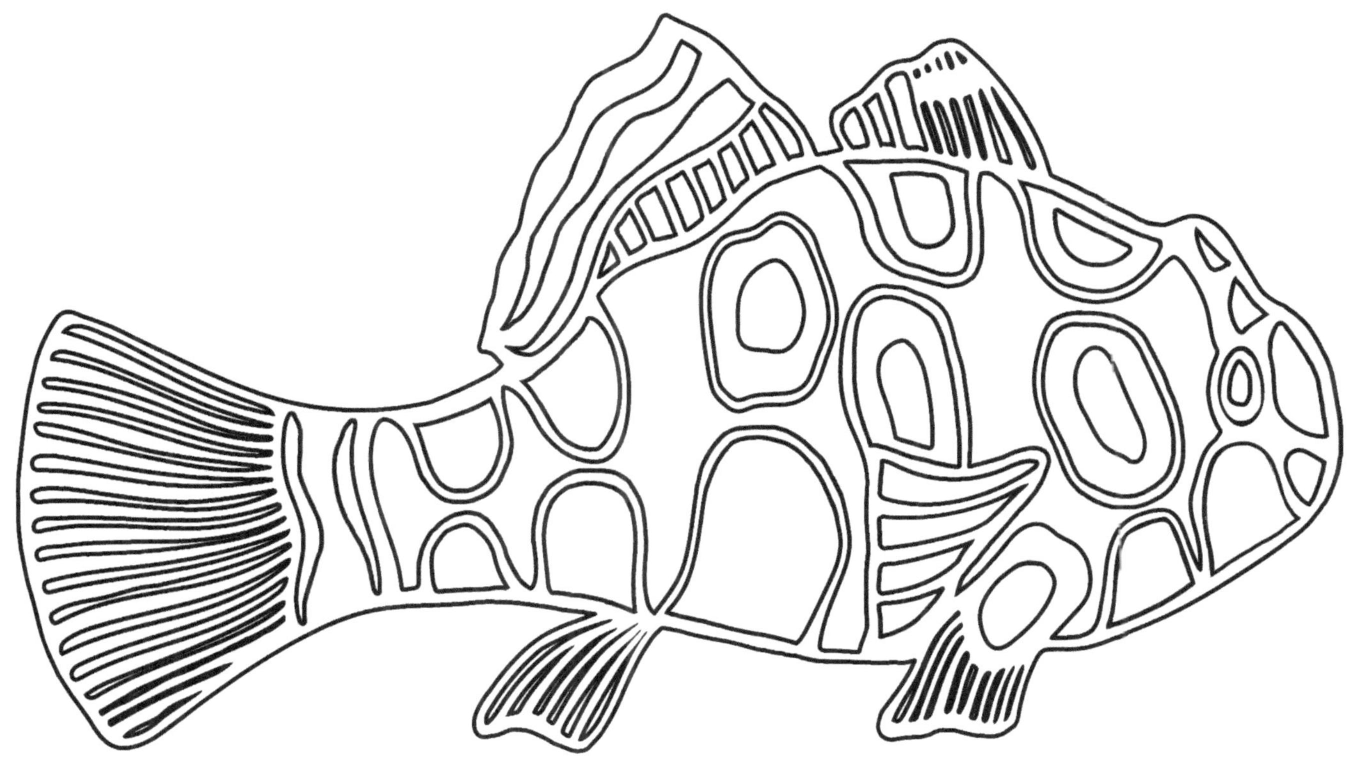

Trust Me

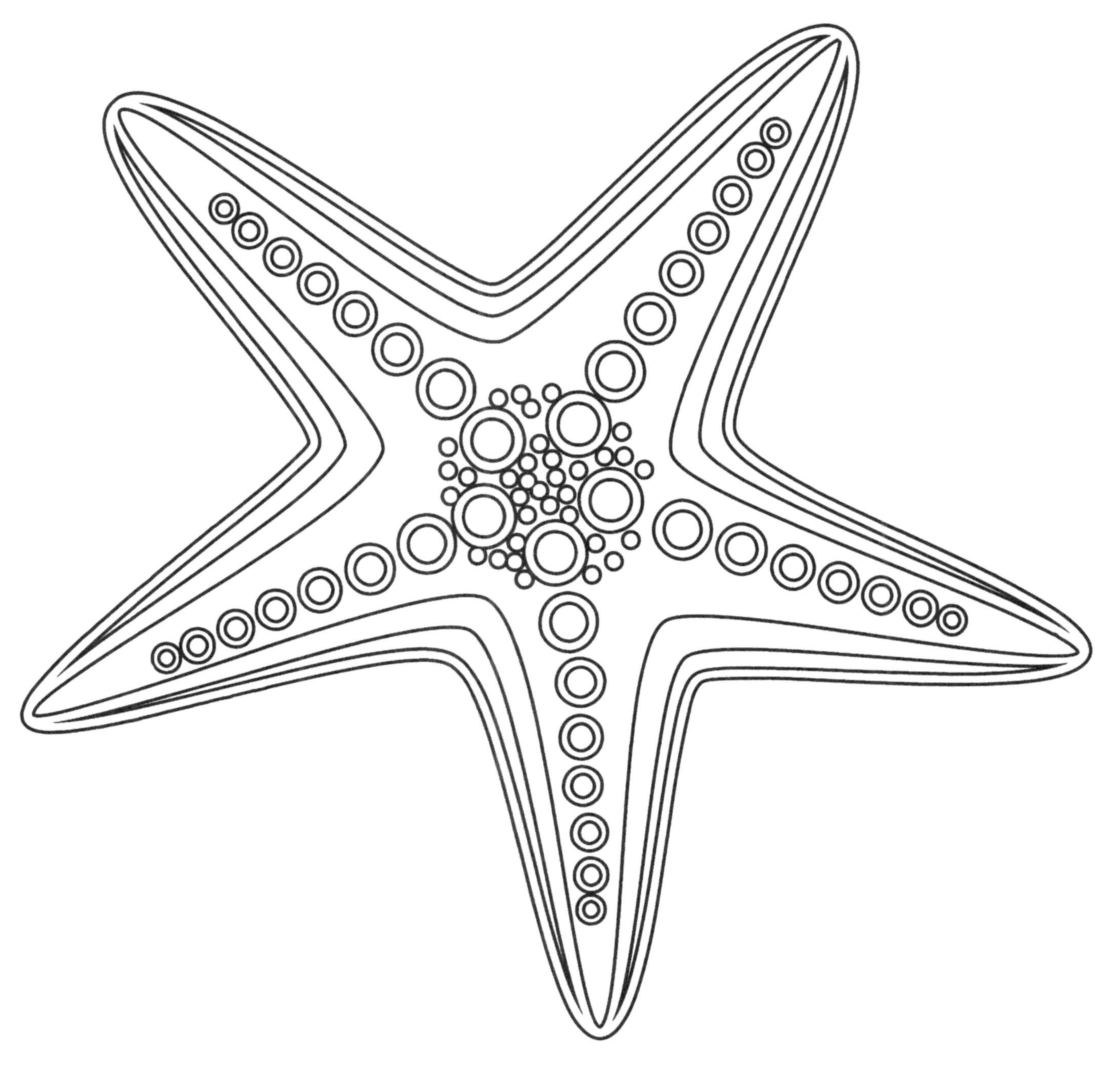

Try Again

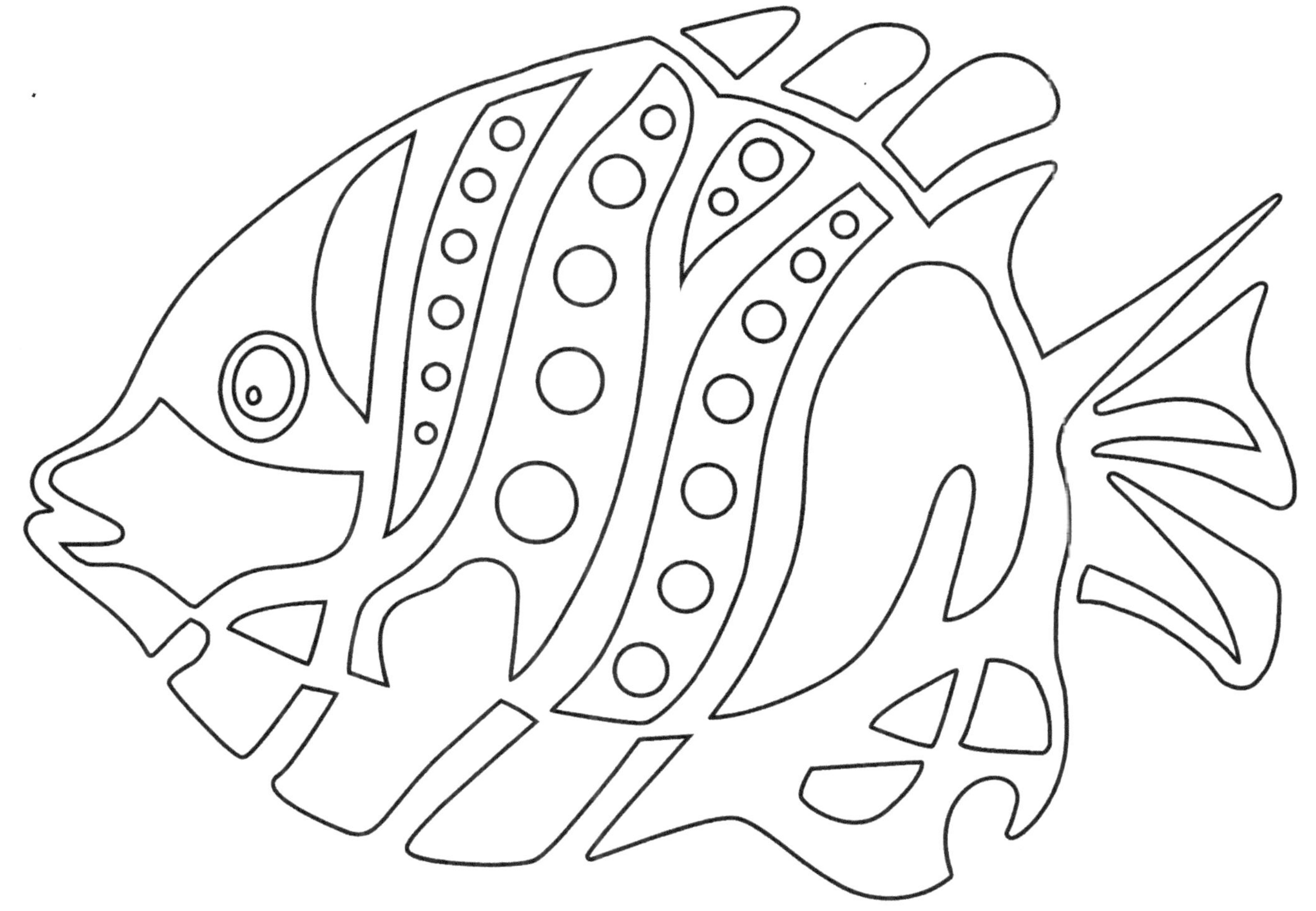

You Can

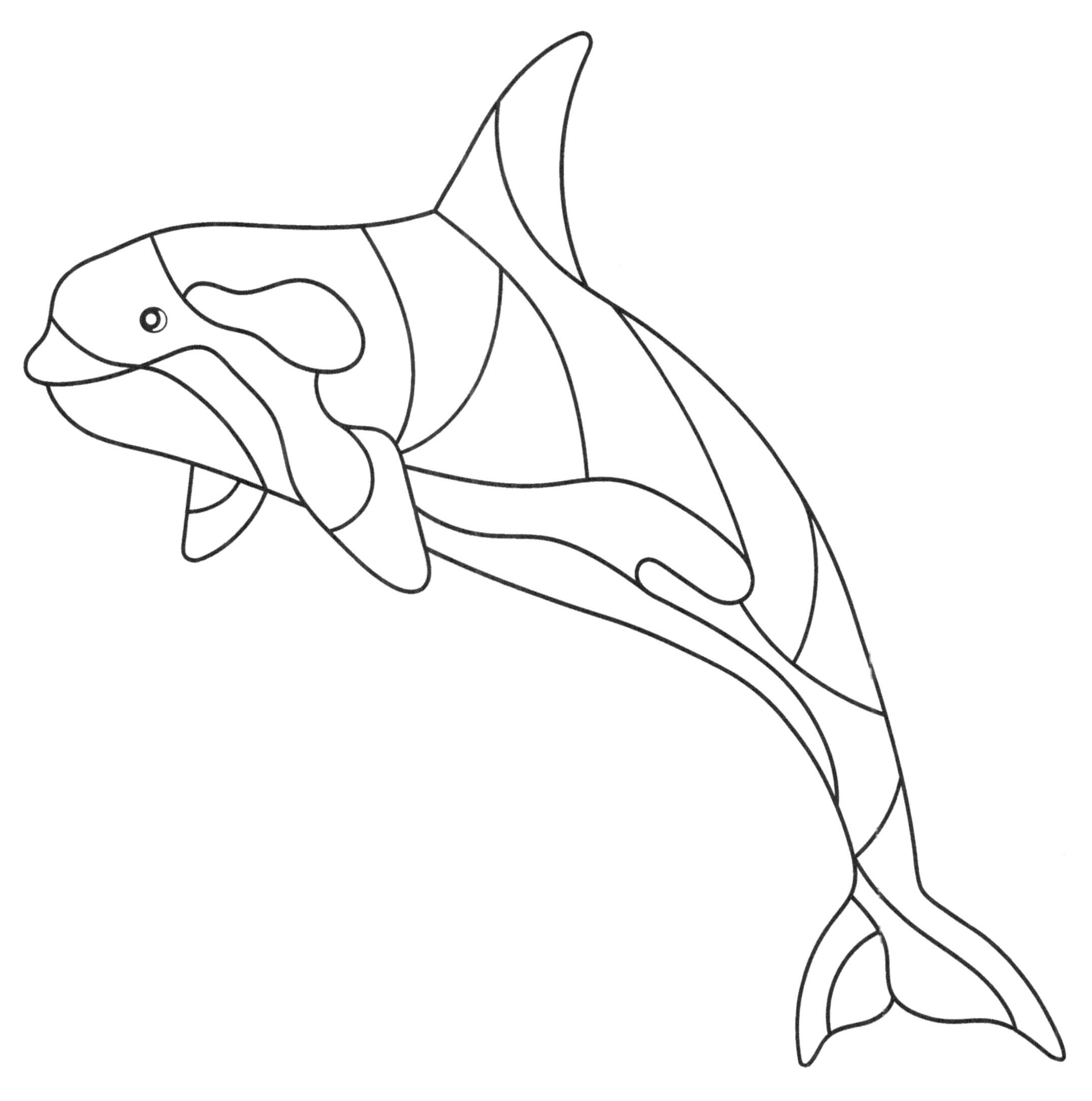

You Matter

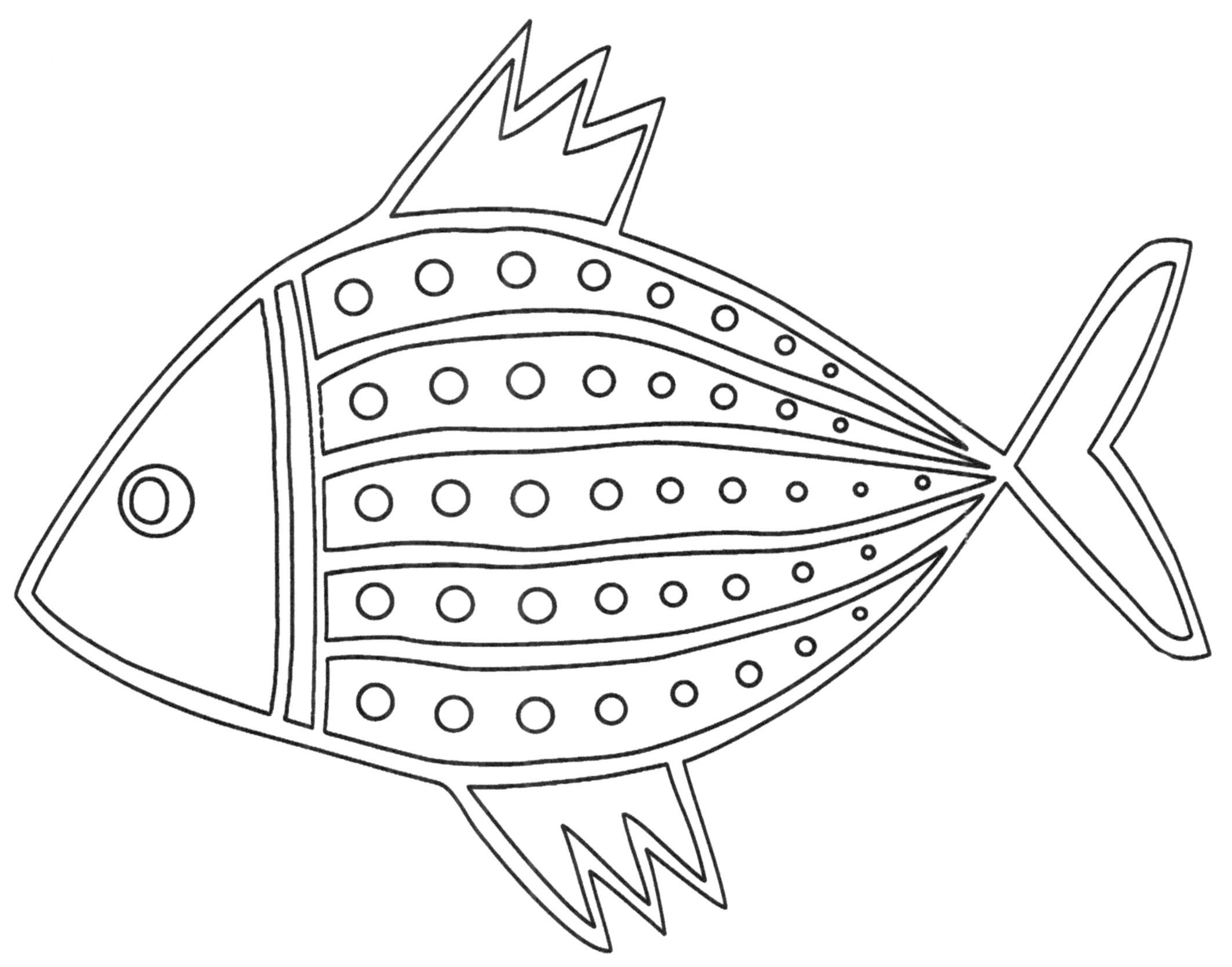

You're Blessed